"There is no more important mission today than to coach people who are struggling and want to improve their health and wellness. Bob Merberg is among the first to embrace this mission, and has become a founding father of health and wellness coaching. I have no doubt that the wisdom and advice in *The Health Seeker's Handbook* will stand the test of time. It's my great privilege to be associated with Bob."

———Margaret Moore
Founder and CEO, Wellcoaches Corporation
www.wellcoaches.com

"Bob Merberg is like a sailboat tacking back and forth across your mind, discovering the wind to get you to your goal. Perceptive and encouraging, he assisted me in setting realistic goals without the words *should* or *must*. He can help you reach your objective and beyond."

———Palmeda Day, R.N.

"Bob Merberg's *The Health Seeker's Handbook* takes a refreshing step out of the stressful minutiae of typical health advice. Rather, it focuses on the big picture, the whole person, in a way you can live with day to day."

———Will Clower, Ph.D.
author, *The Fat Fallacy*

"In *The Health Seeker's Handbook*, Bob Merberg demonstrates remarkable insight into the internal obstacles that stand in the way of behavioral change. And he has a rare capacity to guide people around those obstacles, and sometimes right through them."

———Dennis Glick, M.D.
Certified Professional in Health Care Quality

H^{THE}EALTH
SEEKER'S
HANDBOOK

THE
HEALTH
SEEKER'S
HANDBOOK

Revolutionary Advice on How to
Shape Up, Trim Down, and Chill Out
from America's #1 Health Coach

BOB MERBERG

Well Lit Books
East Amherst, New York

Well Lit Books
8677 Millcreek Drive
East Amherst, NY 14051

Copyeditor: Lucy Gardner Carson
Cover layout: Michael Anthony Lynch
Interior design: John Culleton
Author photo: Sharon Campagna
Cover art: Warren Bellows

ISBN 0-9743762-4-8
Manufactured in the United States of America
Library of Congress Card Number: 2003110378
The information contained in this book is not intended to replace the advice of a physician or other health-care professional. Any use of the information in this book is at the reader's discretion. The author and publisher cannot be held responsible for any error, omission, professional disagreement, outdated material, or adverse outcomes that may be derived from use of any of the strategies described herein. A health-care professional should be consulted regarding your specific situation.

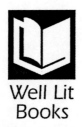

Well Lit
Books

For my dad

CONTENTS

ACKNOWLEDGMENTS

My deepest gratitude goes to Barbara Clarke, who opened my eyes to the world of coaching, the world of publishing, and the world at large. I am humbled by her friendship.

In many respects, this book is the brainchild of the various teachers with whom I have been fortunate enough to cross paths over the course of my life—George Rubino, who was among the first to encourage me to write, and who I heard time and time again urging students to "write it as you would say it"; the late John C. Gardner, who honored me with his musings on writing and on life; Master Hidy Ochiai, really my first coach, who brought out my best and instilled in me a passion for harmony of mind and body; Ven. Thich Nhat Hanh, whose teachings on mindfulness and loving-kindness have shaped me and this book; Rev. Joel Miller, whose humor, wonder, and wisdom help sustain me; and Jack Kornfield, from whom I learned that the running commentary in my mind is delightfully ordinary.

I extend a virtual thank-you hug to the entire teaching staff at Coach U, especially Bobette Reeder, whose "want" for me prompted my discovery of a new possibility; Rachel Disbennett-Lee, who "had a feeling" about my success as a coach; and Phyliss Wolf, who accepted me as is and showed me unprecedented support. And I thank Thomas Leonard, the founder of Coach U and of the coaching profession as a whole, who died unexpectedly as I was completing this book. I learned much from Thomas during our brief collaboration, not the least of which was to "eliminate delay"—a classic Thomas distillation that still brings a smile to my face.

I offer my heartfelt thanks to a circle of extraordinary professionals with whom I shared a ride on the health-care Tilt-a-Whirl: Jeanie Young, R.N., whose commitment to quality and to a loving style of leadership profoundly influenced my coaching; Cindan Gizzi, M.P.H., who modeled for me how to bring creative brilliance to health promotion; and Dave Huyg, who stood by my side (and usually carried the load) through endless health fairs and self-care workshops. I thank Jana Pinkerton, R.D., Cathy Lumb-Edwards, Janet Johnson-Yosgott, and Michelle Carnahan, M.P.H., a dream team of health educators who offered me not only their friendship, but their humor, their kindness, and their wisdom; and Jill Nussinow, R.D., who helped me find joy in healthful eating and gave me sage publishing advice at the place I least expected it—under the blue light at a K-Mart in Santa Rosa, California. One never knows where gifts will appear.

Lucy Gardner Carson came to me as a copyeditor, but delivered so much more—adopting this publishing project in its nascence and holding it as if it were her own. I marvel at the good fortune of having Lucy on my team.

I thank Dennis Glick, M.D., whose "slap therapy" opened the door for me to build my coaching practice and to write this book and whose receptivity provided the validation I needed when the going got tough; and Warren Bellows, who, when he wasn't inserting needles into my feet or scalp, needled my point of view.

I am forever indebted to my father and my late mother. This book could not have been written had I not been blessed with their unconditional and everlasting support.

ACKNOWLEDGMENTS

As a coach and as a writer, I have been nourished and emboldened by my brother, David, and my sister, Elinor. I'm so glad that, as kids, they turned a deaf ear when chided, "Don't encourage him."

For their unequivocal confidence in me, I thank Margaret Moore, Sheryl Marks Brown, Arnie Freiman, Ph.D., Bonnie Story, Donna Lockhart, R.N., Mary Stein, A.N.P., Polly Day, R.N., Barbara Graves, Sean Slovenski, Diane Tapogna, R.N., John Baxter, Vanessa Bryson, and my many cherished clients, from whom, over the years, I have learned so much about health change and about myself.

Finally, my deep and loving thanks goes to my wife, Eileen—my salvation—who has not wavered for a second as I travel this tenuous journey of coaching and writing. And to our faithful children, Oren and Maya: Thank you for putting up with Daddy as he frittered away all that time—*your* time—on the computer and on the phone. My love for you is boundless.

Introduction

KICK THE WILLPOWER HABIT

You choose the actions that affect your health—but *choice* does not depend on *willpower.* In fact, blind devotion to willpower as a panacea for unwanted health habits can ensnare you like a rabid bulldog chomping down on your ankle, pulling you away from your ultimate destination, refusing to set you free no matter how wildly you thrash about.

When you do successfully adopt healthy new behaviors or drop unhealthy old ones, it won't be by out-willing your desires; it will be by redirecting them. You'll establish a sense of ease so that you instinctively choose self-care over self-destruction. And, as you read this book, you'll be bolstered by individualized coaching strategies that have been proven to evoke successful change. This is the organic process for health change, and it works. In my experience as a health educator, fitness trainer, and personal health coach, I have found it to be the only process that *does* work.

Most seekers of better health steadfastly adhere to their dependence on willpower. Perhaps it's the "rugged individual" model with which many of us are raised that leads us to buy into this willpower legend. Yet willpower rarely plays anything more than a supporting role in health change. The very words "will" and "power" set health seekers up for a struggle. Positive health change, however, results not from the adversarial forces inside you, but from your constructive qualities, including confidence, joy, self-respect, and courage. The sooner you can loosen the grip willpower has over you, the sooner you will make whatever health change you wish to make.

What's the alternative to willpower? When I coach health seekers—guiding them in periodic telephone sessions through a

3

process of *goal setting, strategic planning,* and *self-discovery*—they consistently make three specific underlying shifts that set their behavioral change in motion:

1. They *Shape Up* their lives, by discovering new possibilities, increasing their confidence, creating an environment that's conducive to healthy living, establishing strong supportive relationships, and building on their strengths.

2. They *Trim Down* their distractions, by tuning in their self-awareness, simplifying their lifestyles, letting go of stale goals, clarifying and focusing on what's truly important to them, and being fully present in the moment.

3. They *Chill Out,* by taking leave of guilt, disappointment, limiting beliefs, and other forms of self-deprecation that stand in the way of well-being.

I call these shifts the underpinnings of change. They support the successful transformation of what we've come to think of as bad health habits—unhealthful eating, insufficient exercise, unmanaged stress, smoking, and so forth.

The Health Seeker's Handbook includes all the strategies you need to shape up, trim down, and chill out, and beyond that, to change your daily health habits once and for all.

This is not a weight-loss book, though it can help you lose weight if that's what you're after. It's not a fitness book, though it can guide you to peak performance with a lot less effort. And it's not a stress-reduction book, though by following the advice on these pages, you will more easily adopt stress-reduction techniques (and have a lot less stress in your life to begin with).

Health is the focus here; but as you will see, you can delve much deeper than that. Strategies for change tend to be similar for most aspects of your lifestyle—your career, your patterns of dealing with relationships, and your personal financial management, to name a few. Indeed, you'll soon see that all of these may be considered facets of what we call health.

A Zero-Step Plan

Bookstore shelves are overflowing with self-help manuals about how to fix whatever ails you with such-and-such six-week program or So-and-So's twenty-five-step plan. But in reality there is no formula that will work for each and every seeker of health.

In *The Health Seeker's Handbook,* I offer you a zero-step plan as an alternative. The idea is that if you are serious about living a healthier lifestyle, you have to find your own path. This is why I use the term "health seeker": You seek true solutions, not just mass-marketed hype or easy answers.

It's your life and your health. The challenges that present themselves to you, as well as the strengths and resources available to you, are unique—your health-change fingerprint, of sorts. Trying to cram a mass-marketed program into your life—or, as is more often the case, cramming your life into a program—is exactly what this book is *not* about.

What you will find here, rather than a *formula* for success, are the *elements* of success, based on the latest research and on my experience with thousands of health seekers. You will learn the strategies, tactics, procedures, outlooks, tips, and techniques that define success. It's up to you to sift through these elements—deciding which ones you'll use, which ones you'll discard, and how much time you'll take—because, as the resident of your own body, you are uniquely qualified to do so.

This will be an exciting yet straightforward path.

Revolutionary Solutions

A few years ago, I launched a biweekly e-mail newsletter called *The Health Coach.* My intention was for each issue to feature a snippet of health-coaching wisdom that readers could use immediately to help them eat healthier, exercise more, reduce stress, or make any lifestyle change that would bring them a greater sense of well-being. I promised readers that *The Health Coach* would shun the same old song and dance they might see in health magazines or hear from other health professionals.

The Health Coach integrated the most successful coaching methods with the best proven conventional approaches. It offered revolutionary solutions for readers vexed with the dilemma *"I know what to do to lose weight [or eat better, or exercise, or quit smoking], but I just can't get myself to do it."* In essence, each snippet described one of the elements associated with profound and lasting health change.

When *The Health Coach* first launched, it had thirty subscribers, many of whom were my own friends, family, and existing clients. Within a year, word had spread and the subscriber list had ballooned to 2,200—reaching readers in more than fourteen countries worldwide.[1]

During this period, I was incubating The Center for Personal Health Coaching—an online resource center. Meanwhile, I was

---

[1] *The Health Coach* continues to grow by approximately 1,000 subscribers annually; you can subscribe any time at: www.healthcoach4u.com.

deluged with e-mails from subscribers who had experienced a dramatic improvement in their well-being, sometimes as a result of one particular issue of the newsletter; more frequently as a result of their own individual concoction of various health-change elements I presented to them over time. You now hold in your hands a complete collection of these elements, and you can reap the same rewards.

Most of the guidance in this book is loosely based on the three underpinnings of change: shaping up, trimming down, and chilling out. But this is not an exact science; and really, it's not important what goes where. This is a true *handbook:* The elements are presented for you to pick and choose, mix and match.

A word of advice: For each element in the handbook, I have included a related activity under the heading "Mind Your Change." These represent real requests—homework assignments, if you will—that at times I make of my coaching clients. When you discover an element that appeals to you (and sometimes even if it doesn't), do the activity. "Mind Your Change" activities were developed specifically to assist you in shifting your health change from an *idea* to an *action.* If the activity instructs you to write a list or talk to a peer about something, then *do it*—don't just *think* of the list or imagine the conversation in your head. The object here is to get your health change out of your head (so it's not just an idea) and into the physical world (so you're taking action). Your idea to change, when residing only in your head, is like an eagle's egg in the nest—raw potential. Our goal is to nurture that idea, hatch it, teach it to fly, and send it soaring out into the world.

What Is Health? And Who Really Cares?

Prior to the 1940s, the word "health" was commonly defined as the absence of disease. In 1948, the World Health Organization (WHO) offered a new definition of health: a state of complete physical, social, and mental well-being. Nearly forty years later, the European section of WHO went even further and proclaimed that health is:

> ...the extent to which an individual or group is able on the one hand to realize aspirations and satisfy needs, and, on the other hand, to change and cope with the environment. Health is therefore seen as a resource for everyday life, not the objective of living. It is a positive concept emphasizing social and personal resources as well as physical capacities. *(Ottawa Charter for Health Promotion, 1986)*

In the latter half of the twentieth century, the concept of "wellness" was introduced. Wellness, as originally defined, meant a state of being in which health seekers achieve maximal potential in the physical, emotional, psychological, and spiritual dynamics of life and live in such a way that helps them continuously uncover new potential.

I note these definitions only to encourage you to re-evaluate your own vision of health. Personally, I use the words "wellness," "well-being," and "health" interchangeably. But for your purposes, it doesn't matter what these concepts mean to me or to some researcher. I do not purport to help you achieve what I or anyone else believes health to be, but to show you the way to achieve health as *you* define it, on your own terms.

In this book, I cite plenty of examples related to fitness, eating, weight management, and stress, because those are common areas of concern these days. But if health to you means, say, watching less TV or getting to the beach more frequently, you will still find in *The Health Seeker's Handbook* strategies that get you to your goal.

I view your time as precious, so I do not squander it or insult your intelligence harping on the little health habits you should adopt—the foods you should eat, the kind of exercise you need, the components of stress management. You already know this stuff, and if you don't, you have countless resources available to you—media, classes, friends, health professionals, your mom, and so forth. *The Health Seeker's Handbook* offers something new and practical: It shows you how to do what you know you need (or want) to do. Where appropriate, I have described the more progressive and effective techniques for getting fit, losing weight, and reducing stress, especially those that, to some extent, reflect a coaching approach. But these do not constitute the crux of this collection, because they are worthless to you until you identify focused, proven strategies for catalyzing successful and permanent change, such as those offered here.

How to Scale a Brick Wall

I haven't always been a personal health coach. I worked for fifteen years or so as a health educator, wellness professional, lecturer, and personal trainer, fruitlessly trying to prod people into better health using all the old tricks: setting goals, having clients sign contracts with themselves, and offering trite incentives, such as water bottles and insulated lunch bags. I found that in most cases this conventional approach—what I call health behaviorism—didn't work. Inevitably, clients grew discouraged, bored, or just flat-out disgusted with having to shoehorn into their hectic lives new, "healthy" habits that were completely out of sync with their personalities. What's more, health-seeking humans, unlike cheese-seeking rats or thirsty canines, cleverly and effectively resist being manipulated by simple rewards.

Unwilling to resign myself to the idea that people can't change, I increasingly restructured my interventions with health seekers. I spent less time trying to manipulate them and more time listening to what was really standing in their way. Soon I realized that most health seekers were running up against brick walls that our conventional approaches never fully addressed. The most common ones:

- Most health seekers don't have time to add new health habits to everything they already are doing in their lives. Traditionally, health educators might address this by offering help with time management. But such an approach overlooks the fact that it's not just the health seekers' perceptions— they genuinely *don't* have enough time.

- Many health seekers don't have the energy to adopt new behaviors. They're exhausted.

- Often, health seekers can't conceive of themselves living differently for the remainder of their lives.

- Attempts at health change are profoundly influenced by other people. Health seekers need proactive support from others in their lives, yet their efforts are often undermined by loved ones (sometimes intentionally, sometimes inadvertently).

- Health seekers tend to have an unwavering belief that the key to their success is strong willpower. This is accompanied by their belief that their own willpower is not strong enough to make a permanent change. Their efforts are reduced to a war of the wills—in this case, a civil war, executed on the landscape of the health seeker's own heart and mind. Success is inevitably the casualty of this war of the wills. Guilt, shame, and negative self-talk are the heavy artillery.

While conventional health-behavior strategies target a few of these issues, I know of none that addresses them all, and none that addresses them boldly and holistically. That's where coaching comes in.

Recall that coaching is a process in which a trained coach guides clients through a process of goal setting, strategizing, and self-discovery, and notice that there are commonalities between coaching and health behaviorism: For example, goal setting is intrinsic to both. On the other hand, few nutritionists or personal fitness trainers are trained or comfortable in the arena of self-discovery. Yet self-discovery is at the heart of coaching. With a coach as facilitator, motivator, and guide, the client identifies his own goals, his own obstacles, and his own solutions (which, as a natural result of this process, are completely individualized).

Health behaviorism *does* have much to offer; it is foolhardy to dismiss it. Coaching and health behaviorism complement each other. But even with the strengths of these two approaches, something is still missing.

It's All in Your Mind

Ultimately, when someone wants to make a lasting health change, nothing short of personal transformation is required. The coaching industry boasts that personal transformation is its end result, and that's true to an extent. But, as you well know, changing health habits is a precipitous enterprise. It requires a solution more profound and more potent than typical coaching methods provide.

As a health coach, I incorporate health behavioral strategies and coaching techniques, but the fuel for lasting change is yet something else: *mindfulness*—raw attention to the present moment. Mindfulness is not derived from coaching or from behaviorism, but from ancient wisdom. In the past twenty years, mindfulness has been incorporated as a healing modality, and its value has been well documented.

Mindfulness, coaching, and behaviorism: Within the integration of these three realms lie the art and science of health change.

I Believe in You

When I first wrote these pieces for *The Health Coach,* I did so quite intuitively, thinking of subscribers as my coaching clients. I strove to make the reading compelling and sometimes humorous, and I struck the same tone I would have if I were speaking to a client one on one. I have preserved that style in this handbook, because I believe it's a big part of why *The Health Coach* newsletter has been so successful: Readers readily come to feel like my coaching clients, like they know me and I know them. Our relationship is so strong largely because, rather than presenting myself as the world's foremost authority on life, as many health and self-help authors are prone to do, I recognize that I, too, am a health seeker. I have been on this path for a long time, with my fair share of both victories and setbacks, and I understand—better than any buffed-up fitness guru or celebrity health spokesperson ever will—what makes health seekers tick and how best to help them.

I encourage you to think of yourself as my client, too. My priority has always been to treat readers with the respect, honesty, and earnestness with which I treat my clients, and with which my own coaches (and clients) have treated me. It is in this relationship, based on mutual truthfulness and openness, that the power of coaching lies. So open up and grant yourself permission to join this relationship right now.

I believe in you. Each individual is full of potential, each individual is coachable, and you should never resign yourself to believing that you are unable to do what you want to do. You *are* able. If at any point, however, you *choose* not to pursue your goal, then that choice is yours. You are not the victim of nature, or nurture, or anything else. If you achieve your goal— be it weight loss, or fitness, or stress reduction—I celebrate you. And if you elect not to lose weight, or not to exercise more, or not to reduce stress... that is your choice, too. I will not judge you, nor should anyone else. And I still will celebrate you.

Welcome!

Part I
Shape Up

DISCOVER YOUR POSSIBILITY

I DON'T know if the story about Christopher Columbus is true, but even as a legendary figure he was an inspiring case. It's understandable that, back then, most people thought the world was flat. But Columbus—using scientific observation and a good dose of intuition, and probably listening to some smart friends—envisioned a world far beyond what his senses could perceive.

You can do the same thing in your world. Find the unlimited potential. Discover the possibility of who you are or can be—far beyond what you ordinarily perceive as possible.

When I ask my new clients what has stirred them to reach new heights in their lives, they usually tell me it was their *vision of a possibility* for themselves. Often, the seed of this possibility was planted in them by someone else who could see their potential much more clearly than they themselves could see it.

In my coaching practice, I help health seekers discover new possibilities for themselves. At first glance, their vision of who they can become may be limited, as a result of the social environments in which they have lived. Consequently, they set goals that tend to be less than inspiring.

But when I tell a health seeker who has been sedentary for ten years that within a year she can walk a marathon, or ride a bicycle all the way up the coast, that really gets her going! It is the promise of transformation that ultimately lights us up. The sedentary health seeker who pictures herself crossing the finish line of a marathon knows that, under those circumstances, she will be thinking, acting, and living as a renewed person. And *that's* a goal with a long lifespan.

When I first started coaching, I had difficulty helping weight-loss clients discover their possibilities. What would I say? "Janet, you are going to be so successful with your weight loss that some day you won't weigh anything at all"? I don't think so.

But over time, I learned to dig deeper with these clients. Often, I came to use a simple technique I call "Digging Up the Roots." This is a method of excavating a client's possibility (it also can be used to effectively drill down on obstacles) by making the almost childlike inquiry, "Why?" until we have reached the root of the matter.

A typical Digging Up the Roots conversation with a weight-loss client occurred with a health seeker I'll call Amelia:

Coach: "Why do you want to lose weight, Amelia?"

Amelia: "So I can look better."

Coach: "Why do you want to look better?"

Amelia: "So I feel better about myself."

Coach: "Why do you want to feel better about yourself?"

Amelia: "I think people will like me more if I feel better about myself."

Coach: "Why do you want people to like you more?"

Amelia: "So I have a lot of friends."

Coach: "Why do you want a lot of friends?"

Amelia: "I'm afraid that as I get older, I'm going to be all alone. I'm afraid of growing old alone and of dying alone."

Now we've gotten somewhere.

For Amelia, the possibility was to be self-confident and to have a vibrant and enduring social life, with a wide network of friends and family contacts. She wanted to feel like she belonged and, as it turned out, she also wanted to feel needed. Many of Amelia's needs stemmed from her fear of aging.

Don't get me wrong: Amelia's weight-loss goal was not dismissed. As long as she believed her weight interfered with her self-esteem and her social life, it would. Some health seekers might be more inclined to shift these beliefs rather than focus on the outcome. But Amelia had her heart set on weight loss, and as she confronted the challenges of that elusive goal, she was bolstered by the image of herself as a self-confident, ebullient person with a strong connection to others. Her fear of aging naturally abated as her vision of the future brightened. And ultimately, Amelia's possibility became her reality.

As you can see, possibility doesn't always simply appear in front of you. Sometimes you have to do some exploring, just as Columbus did. After all, old Chris didn't just look out his window and say, "Whoa! I guess the earth *is* flat!" He went out to take a look-see for himself.

In rare cases, the first possibility you conjure up may be something that is physically impossible. This is another instance when Digging Up the Roots comes in handy. For example, my client Roger was a former skier who had injured his knee, and his doctors warned him not to ski again. Knee pain had now become a part of his life. When he first hired me, he felt like his enthusiasm for exercise and for staying in top shape was starting to wane. Roger was a great explorer of possibility. He not only dreamed of being an elite skier, and of being in the Winter Olympics, but really he wanted to win a gold medal! Well, he had never skied at that level—which isn't to say that he never could have. But with his injured knee, it really wasn't going to happen, and to suggest otherwise would have encouraged Roger to endure a lot of pain for no reason and probably to ruin his knee and his life.

When Roger and I dug up the roots, he discovered that, more than anything, he wanted to be the best. He wanted recognition, and he wanted to test his limits.

Roger now sees himself as the ultimate 100-yard freestyle record-holder for his age group in Masters Swimming. And he is well on his way to realizing this possibility.

In our culture, we generally find it easy to help our children discover possibilities. When we say, "Someday, you could be president of the United States," or "Someday, you could play for the Yankees," we are shining a light on their possibility. Sadly, as people get older they tend to shine this light less readily for others, partially because they themselves may be growing blind to the possibilities.

But in my own case, I am being authentic when I help clients discover their possibilities. I hold a steadfast belief in the unlimited potential of each and every health seeker, just as I hold a steadfast belief in my own possibility. And in yours.

MIND YOUR CHANGE

Dig up the roots of your biggest health goal. Why do you want to attain this goal? When you answer "x," ask "Why do I want x?" and so forth. Sometimes it will take five why's or fewer, sometimes more, to get to the root. But you'll know it when you get there. Write your answers in a journal or on any piece of paper, and then write, in as much detail as you can imagine, your possibility for yourself. How will it feel to be you once you have *become* your possibility?

Try this exercise again with your primary work goal, relationship goal, or financial goal. You may find that the possibilities you discover from these goals share the same root you dug up at the base of your health goal. More often than not, health seekers' various life goals sprout from the same source.

The Write Way to Health

Even if you've never thought of yourself as the "journaling type," keep a daily journal when you're striving to change a health habit. You'll be amazed at what a difference it can make for you.

Health seekers often feel stuck because their health goals are nothing more than ideas in their mind. Their task at hand is to shake those ideas loose and transform them into *actions*.

One of the many benefits of journaling is that it serves as an idea shaker. As you journal about your thoughts, feelings, and perceptions around your health change, you facilitate an exchange between your internal and external worlds, and in doing so you break through toward action. To get this flow started (or to keep it going), your journaling doesn't have to be specifically about your health change. You can journal about whatever comes to mind.

Use any medium for your journal: a nice bound book, a computer, or even a tape recorder—whatever you are most comfortable with. But don't delay your journaling until you find the perfect medium. That's a common trap for new journalers: They hunt for the finest, most meaningful journal, until their enthusiasm for the whole thing wanes and is forgotten. *Start today*—on a paper napkin if necessary.

Don't worry about the content of your journal; just let your pen (or your typing fingers) flow. But if you draw a blank, get things rolling with some simple entries about your health change. Consider writing about:

- Achievements you've had in the past twenty-four hours.

- Any challenges you encounter.

- Opportunities that are presenting themselves.

- Lessons learned.

- Feelings, perceptions, and thoughts about how things are going.

- Goals for the next twenty-four hours.

If the process doesn't flow for you, or you simply find that you don't like writing in your journal, don't give up. You may wish to re-examine your idea of what a journal is. There is nothing that *should* or *should not* be entered in a journal. Have fun with it! I encourage clients who keep handwritten journals to use colored pencils when they make entries and to include illustrations, as well. Some clients select colors that fit their moods; others choose arbitrarily. I also suggest that they consider pasting media clippings into their journals, or including business cards of unusual people they've met or greeting cards from loved ones. When my clients review past entries in their journals (for those who do; some choose never to look back), they see a colorful, eclectic record of their lives.

Journaling can be fun, beautiful, and full of joy, and there is no end to the ways in which it will reinforce your health change. For example, it serves as a self-coaching tool. One of the main reasons personal coaching is so effective is because clients feel accountable to their coach. When they set goals and know they are going to be "reporting in" their results, they feel extra motivation to achieve those goals. But ultimately, you are accountable only to yourself. And as you enter your goals and your results in your journal, you are in effect reporting in to yourself. Then, if you define in your journal the circumstances around your outcomes and strategize accordingly, you are acting as your own coach—something you can do for the rest of your life.

Journal your way to better health.

MIND YOUR CHANGE

Today, start journaling about your health change. Don't feel obligated to make entries of any particular length. Not in the mood? No time? Fine. At least enter *one sentence*. Or even one word! But make an entry every day. Commit to this for two weeks. Then, if you don't feel a desire to continue . . . no problem, you can stop. But most likely you will be astonished at where this little exercise takes you.

POWER-UP HEALTH CONFIDENCE: THREE KEY STRATEGIES

Ever wonder why some people can successfully make health changes while others fall short? One of the key factors is what I call *health confidence.* Health confidence is your belief in your own ability to make a health change. It's the difference between *"I'm going to make this change and nothing's going to stop me!"* versus *"I don't know if I can do it, but I'll try."*

Two important things to understand about health confidence:

1. Health confidence is behavior specific; that is, you can be super-confident in your ability to, say, exercise five days a week, but have zero confidence that you can eat healthier.

2. Health confidence can be fostered; you're not stuck at your current level.

It's this latter point that is really critical. As you endeavor to transform your own health, you need to know that your confidence can be boosted. Don't resign yourself to low confidence.

Here are the three key strategies to give your health confidence a lift:

1. *Identify role models.* Seek out people who have already made the change you're trying to make. They will inspire you.

2. *Get cheerleaders.* As much as possible, surround yourself with people who will give you unconditional support, who will celebrate your milestones, and who will help you up if you fall down. This is where a good coach can work

wonders, but if you look around you'll also find friends, family, coworkers, and support groups who will eagerly serve in this role.

3. *Practice.* Tried to make this change before? Don't view previous attempts as a string of failures—they're not. View them as valuable steps toward success. Each step affords you lessons about potential pitfalls and brings you closer to your ultimate goal. Also, think about other positive changes you've made in your life, and be your own role model.

I didn't invent the idea of health confidence. It's based on theories of self-efficacy developed and researched by noted Stanford psychologist Albert Banduras. And there's a wide body of evidence proving that these strategies work.

Three strategies that are easy and that work. What more could you ask for? Why not put them into play today and power-up *your* health confidence?

MIND YOUR CHANGE
Write a list of ten successful health changes, big or small, that you've made in your life. Can't think of ten? What about switching to lower-fat milk, eating less meat, flossing, or drinking more water (these are just some ideas)? What factors in your life facilitated those successes?

THE PERILS OF POSITIVE THINKING

HEALTH confidence is not to be confused with the power of positive thinking. Don't get me wrong: Positive thinking is beneficial. But it must be executed skillfully and discriminately. Otherwise, it just may backfire.

The most important thing about positive thinking is to direct it toward those outcomes that are under your control. So, yes, you must believe that you *will* eat healthier, exercise regularly, floss every day, or gain balance in your work and family life, if those are things you want to do. But these days, positive thinking seems to have taken on a whole new dimension: People actually believe that they must *think* they'll win the lottery in order to actually win it. I hate to break the news to these well-meaning folk (okay, you caught me: I love to break the news to them), but they probably will not win the lottery. Those are the odds, plain and simple.

If you question whether there are any true perils to chronic positive thinking, you need look no further than Wall Street. How many financial speculators have driven themselves into the ground while feverishly clinging to the hope that a risky investment would reap big rewards? I have witnessed many health seekers doing analogous self-harm as they tenaciously "think positive" about treatments or supplements for weight loss, pain, or even diseases, based solely on misleading marketing messages.

Here are five suggestions to help you frame your positive thoughts so they move you forward, in your health improvement or in any other aspect of your life, rather than hold you back:

1. *Cultivate a positive attitude rather than forcing yourself to think positively.* Attend to the joy of life. For example,

surround yourself with people you love, spend time in nature, or maintain a spiritual connection. Positive thought will naturally follow.

2. *Establish boundaries for your positive thinking.* The media is full of stories about how optimism makes people live longer. Not as well publicized are the countless stories about people who have been bilked out of thousands of dollars as they remained "optimistic" about fraudulent health remedies.

3. *Respect your negative thoughts, and don't try to squelch them with positive thoughts.* Negative thoughts are present in all of us, but they do their most harm when we stuff them so far down into ourselves that we forget they're there. Ultimately, negative thoughts find a way to express themselves, one way or the other.

4. *Identify the silver lining, without distorting the truth.* As a coach, I often help clients see the good in what appears to be a setback. For example, if a client wants to get back the body he had twenty years ago . . . okay, I'll coach him around that. But if a client tells me, "I've resigned myself to the fact that I'll never look like I did twenty years ago," I might offer: "Well, I understand that you feel resigned to that, but another way to look at it is that you've *accepted* it." This type of distinction—from the negative feeling of resignation to the positive feeling of acceptance—will shift a client from thinking he has failed to knowing he has grown.

5. *If your body breaks down or doesn't heal, don't assume it's because you didn't maintain a positive attitude.* Attitudes

affect health, no doubt about it. But sometimes you just get sick or injured. Your body is fallible. And some of the most upbeat people, regrettably, suffer nasty physical ailments.

I'm not a psychotherapist, and I'm not presenting these ideas to you as scientific fact. But over the years, as I have helped thousands of people improve their health, this is what I have known to work.

MIND YOUR CHANGE

In your journal, write a list of 100 things you are grateful for. One hundred may seem like a lot. If you're having a particularly bad day, you may at first not even be able to think of one. But stick with it, and once you get started, you'll be amazed at all the people, places, things, and experiences for which you feel gratitude. You may be thankful to be living during an era when something you love is happening or someone you love is alive. You may be thankful to have certain opportunities or to have seen beautiful scenery. You may be thankful for any or all of your senses or for your health. Perhaps you are thankful for your spiritual faith, for your family, for some talent you have, or just for ever having tasted a cannoli.

Writing your list of 100 gratitudes won't take more than an hour. Yet it is a transformational exercise, well established for cultivating positivism.

ASK AND YE SHALL RECEIVE

I HAVE a darn-near-pathological inability to ask for help, and even greater difficulty accepting help when it is offered, which I have cleverly disguised as "resourcefulness." This was my first big "aha" after I had hired my own coach. As a fieldwork assignment, my coach requested that I ask others for help on at least five occasions during the week to come. She suggested that my request be something as simple as asking a friend to bring me a cup of water, or something bigger, such as requesting a ride to the airport. To my amazement, I was unable to complete the assignment.

These days, I'm better at requesting help, but I still need to work on it. And I find that this challenge has allowed me to more effectively coach some of my own clients who want to develop in this area.

If you're trying to make a big health change, have you requested help from friends, family, or coworkers? Have you graciously accepted and received help when it's been offered? If not, I advise you to do so. Don't go it alone. Having the assistance and support of those around you is likely to be one of the most important conditions for your success. Here are some ideas for requesting help that might fit into your plan:

- Ask a friend to provide moral support.

- If you're trying to become an ex-smoker, ask other smokers not to smoke around you.

- Ask coworkers to take a walk with you. Don't just invite them; *request* it of them.

- Ask your boss for some scheduling flexibility so you can get home earlier to cook a healthier meal, get to a yoga class, or simply spend some quality time with your family.

- Ask your doctor for advice. (Some health seekers are reluctant to request help even from those who are paid to provide it.)

Your ability to receive help correlates closely with your ability to receive other forces that have pull over your well-being. As you tend to this invaluable skill, you will experience a corresponding increase in the adroitness with which you accept into your life both the comforting and the challenging aspects of your environment, your loved ones, and your self.

Gifts surround you all the time. Sometimes you just need to practice receiving them. Learning to receive, I assure you, will bring rewards far beyond physical health.

MIND YOUR CHANGE

You guessed it: On five occasions this week, request help at times when you ordinarily would not. Make the requests as small or as large as you need to in order to stretch your readiness to receive help.

Change Your World

It's ironic that health seekers sometimes think they can do something as challenging and complex as changing a long-held health habit while leaving everything else in their lives the same. For better or worse, it doesn't work like that. In order to change a health habit, you have to change your world. For starters, some simple environmental changes will do. For example:

- If you want to eat healthier, clear your fridge and cupboards of all the unhealthy foods. I'm not going to list what they are here—you know what's not good for you.

- Trying to reduce stress? Create environments that are soothing to you. Use some relaxing aromatherapy, such as lavender or peppermint. Fill your surroundings with soothing music and beautiful pictures of nature or loved ones. Keep some fresh flowers around.

- Getting started with exercise? Manage those aspects of your environment that drain your energy. Eliminate clutter. Complete unfinished projects that are lying around. Do a media fast (a day without use of any kind of media).

Here's another effective approach to changing your world: When you first launch your health change, literally put yourself in a new environment—one that's refreshing and nurturing for you. A spa is great if you can pony up the bucks, but camping in a natural environment or visiting with a supportive family member can also work well.

Ultimately, the bigger the change you're trying to make, the more dramatic will be the environmental modification you need to put into place. So, for example, if you're a smoker trying to quit, stop socializing with other smokers. Does this seem drastic to you? It is. But it's imperative that you do not take any health change too lightly.

And be prepared to change your world.

MIND YOUR CHANGE
We can all stand to lead less stressful lives, at least some of the time. Today, take one action that makes your environment more tranquil. It's so easy, yet well worth doing.

From Resolutions to Real Solutions: Seven Guidelines

I<small>T'S</small> never too early or too late to start thinking about New Year's resolutions. As you read on, you'll understand why. But first, here are seven guidelines you can use to craft New Year's resolutions that stick:

1. *Frame your resolutions in terms of actions, not outcomes.* For example, instead of saying *"I'm going to shape up,"* say *"I will exercise five days a week."* Focus on the steps you are going to take, not just on where they lead. Ideally, weave both into your resolution, as in *"I resolve to shape up by exercising five days a week."*

2. *Be ambitious.* It's okay to start with baby steps, but make sure your resolution challenges and excites you. Here's a subtle, but crucial, distinction: Not *"I'm going to quit cigarettes"*; instead, try *"I'm going to become a nonsmoker."* The first example is about a health behavior, the second, better example is about who you are and how you think of yourself.

3. *But don't be too ambitious.* If you've never exercised, don't resolve to run a marathon every two weeks. But maybe you can walk or run a marathon by the end of the year. Somewhere between an uninspiring resolution and an unrealistic resolution is the perfect resolution for you—one that you can imagine attaining but that is enough of a stretch to keep you fired up.

4. *Make your resolution an intention, not a goal.* The difference? If you don't follow through with an intention, it's no biggie. Perhaps you will another time. Whereas if you don't meet a goal, you're sure to experience guilt and feelings of failure. Does calling your resolution an intention give you permission to slack off? No. You'll give your resolution your best effort, no doubt about it. But, even if the word "intention" doesn't work for you, you must remove the fear of failure. Frankly, fear of failure will only hold you back from making ambitious resolutions.

5. *Accentuate the positive.* Sometimes, health seekers must resolve to *not* do something. Whenever possible, though, try to make your resolution about what you *will* do. Instead of *"I'm going to eat less fatty food,"* go for *"I will eat a [10 percent? 20 percent?] greater proportion of whole-grain foods."*

6. *Quantify.* I guess it's old news, but make your resolutions measurable. Let's say you want to resolve to be less work obsessed. Why? To spend more time with family? To spend more time on your golf game? *"I resolve to limit work to forty hours a week so I can spend at least five more quality hours a week with my family and get my golf score low enough to qualify for the U.S. Open."* Hmmm. That one's not quite there. But it brings us to the final point:

7. *Keep it simple. "I will limit work to forty hours a week and spend at least five more hours with my family."* If you happen to have extra time left over for golf, great. But don't take on too much. My guess is that your family is more important to you than your golf score. If you are single and unattached,

however, have a good day at the links (the golf kind, not the sausage kind).

So, why am I talking about resolutions now? Read the "Mind Your Change" activity that follows.

MIND YOUR CHANGE

Have you composed a New Year's resolution? Good. Now, get started! Why wait? If you have the motivation and the inspiration today, then start today. *Right now.* Stand tall as you demonstrate your commitment to yourself.

Stake Your Claim to Better Health

You have the right to do what you need to do in order to pursue great health. And you have the responsibility to put anyone who might stand in your way on notice that you will not allow their trespasses.

From time to time, friends, spouses, partners, coworkers, bosses, or parents will—to varying degrees—obstruct you, sometimes with the best of intentions and sometimes in order to get their own needs met. They may insist that whatever strategy you have selected doesn't work; try to tempt you into your old patterns of behavior (eating unhealthy food, skipping a workout, and so forth); signal to you, or express outright, their lack of belief in your success; or affect your environment in a manner that is not conducive to self-improvement.

Do not permit this. Standing up for yourself in situations like these not only will eliminate one of the greatest direct threats to your success, but will fill you with the confidence you need to achieve your goal.

Your wellness is yours and yours only. But you must stake your claim. Do not point your finger at others for crossing your boundaries if, indeed, you have not even communicated to them exactly where those boundaries are. Here are some tips for staking your claim and asserting your boundaries:

- *Rely on the spoken word.* If someone is undermining you, you must tell him that he is undermining you, and exactly how he is doing so. This is a good time to use "I" messages about how his actions affect you, such as "I feel unsupported in my effort to lose weight when you keep a lifetime supply of Dove Bars in the freezer."

- *Do not use signals (such as disposing of the Dove Bars), dirty looks, or sarcasm.* You know the difference between good and bad communication. This is no time to be a smart aleck.

- *Be proactive.* If you can anticipate that someone will subvert you, tell her in advance that you will not allow it.

- *Don't be persuaded by the arguments of others that your boundaries may not be reasonable.* Your boundaries are your boundaries. Case closed.

- *Extend your boundaries several steps beyond your comfort zone.* If you're quitting smoking, you may feel like you're setting a boundary by asking your spouse not to smoke in front of you anymore. In fact, you should also tell him not to smoke in the house anymore. Ever. This is the scale upon which you need to be thinking, and acting, in order to make a big-time health change.

MIND YOUR CHANGE

Make a list of five areas of your life in which your boundaries are being crossed. Write an "I" message you can use for each one to stop the trespassing ("*I* feel this way when *you* do such-and-such").

BUILD ON YOUR STRENGTHS

Edith, a fifty-eight-year-old part-time secretary, first hired me as her coach because she was stressed out. Her eighty-five-year-old mother had been living with her since Edith's father had died ten years before, but she had recently admitted her mom into a nursing home because she no longer could provide the necessary intensity of care. No sooner had Edith done this when—lo and behold—her twenty-five-year-old son, Mark, and his wife, Linda, decided that they and their two-year-old daughter, Clarice, needed to move back in with Edith. These young parents had overextended themselves on credit cards and now needed to get back on their feet. And Edith and her husband welcomed them.

Problem was, Mark was working all sorts of hours, and Linda acted as if Edith should share responsibility for the care of the toddler Clarice, though Linda never lifted a finger to clean the house, shop for groceries, or lend a hand in any other way.

Edith's husband did the best he could to help out, doing his part around the house and occasionally making visits to the nursing home when Edith couldn't get there, but he worked, too, and had limited time. Between the two of them, at a stage in their lives when they expected things to be getting easier, things were harder than ever. And the stress was turning Edith into a basket case. She found that the only time she could catch up on her household chores was after everyone else was asleep. Consequently, she was up until midnight every night, and she reported to me that she hadn't had a decent night's sleep in months.

In our early coaching sessions, Edith readily shared an accounting of how her situation was developing and the stress it was causing her, and then tended to steer our conversation toward the safe territory of stress management. At some point, I asked her if she engaged in any kind of regular exercise (one of the most effective stress-management techniques for most people). "Oh, yes," she said. Amazingly, with everything else that was going on, she had still managed to fit in regular exercise. But what I found really remarkable was the *type* of exercise she was doing. "I tried going to the local fitness clubs," she told me, "but it just wasn't my cup of tea. All that glitz and complicated equipment. I took some aerobics classes, but the loud thumping music was very unsettling to me. Then I tried walking, but I didn't like that, either. So finally, I made my own tape of Christian music, and I have my own callisthenic routine that I choreographed to that tape. It takes about thirty minutes, and I do it three times a week. It's a really good workout." Then she slyly added, "Even my daughter-in-law joined in with me once, and she couldn't keep up."

I told Edith that I thought her development of her own exercise routine was pure brilliance. "Edith," I asked. "What personal strengths did you draw upon when you came up with that solution?"

Edith acknowledged that she had drawn upon her strong religious devotion, her discipline, and her determination. I suggested that she also had demonstrated remarkable creative problem-solving skills, self-awareness (she was clear about what she wanted), technical know-how, and thoroughness (exploring all options first and seeing her audiotape project through to completion). I pointed out to her, as well, that she already had demonstrated other strengths to me: a commitment to family, sensitivity, and a strong work ethic, to name a few.

"How can you take these strengths, Edith," I asked at the end of the session, "and use them to not only manage your stress, but to manage your current life situation, so that your stress is reduced by at least 90 percent?"

Over the next few weeks, Edith's life dramatically shifted. She persuaded her daughter-in-law to take little Clarice and visit the nursing home every weekday. Edith still made the visit every chance she got, but this took some pressure off her, while enriching the lives of everyone involved, through four generations in the family. Then, she called a meeting of the entire household and they adopted some rules about sharing chores. In addition, she hired a housecleaner to come in every now and then and had her son's family share the expense (she knew he was strapped for cash but also recognized that part of his recovery could involve accepting more financial responsibility). Eventually, Edith even encouraged her son's family to join her and her husband at the Sunday church service they attended. The invitation was accepted, and the family bond strengthened even further, naturally leading them all, from that point on, to address household problems as a team rather than leaving the load on the shoulders of one person.

While results are not always this dramatic, they often are when health seekers use the coaching approach. In coaching, you *discover* the goal, and you *identify* potential obstacles that stand in the way. Then you *enlist* the resources available to you, especially your personal strengths, to *navigate* those obstacles.

❖

MIND YOUR CHANGE

List your strengths, and decide how you may use them to reach your goal. If you're not sure, consider a goal you have already attained: What strengths did you use in that process? Can some of them be applied to your current endeavor?

CELEBRATE THE ACTION

I'M a big believer in celebrations. It's not that I'm some kind of party animal. But I think that when health seekers make a significant health change, they need to acknowledge themselves every step of the way.

Notice that I said, "every step of the way," and not just at the finish line. By this I mean that you should celebrate your milestones. Usually, health seekers tend to hold off on their celebrations until their ultimate goals have been achieved. They harbor a belief that celebrating a milestone either is overindulgent or will somehow jinx their long-term effort. This is hooey.

Celebrating milestones, even small ones, serves three important purposes:

1. It introduces an element of fun into your plan, which might otherwise feel arduous.

2. It increases your awareness of these milestones, putting them in the limelight when they might otherwise be eclipsed in the shadow of your ultimate goal.

3. It provides continuous motivation.

Usually, I'm in the business of encouraging health seekers to think big. But when it comes to milestones, I urge you to think small. Even minor milestones are worthy of celebrations. So if your long-term goal is to strike a better balance between work and family—say, because you think you've been working too much—then you can celebrate the day you book reservations for your vacation. Don't talk yourself into the idea that the vacation itself is celebration enough. Celebrate the *action*—in this case, booking reservations.

Or, if you are trying to quit smoking, and you visit your physician to learn how to go about it, *celebrate* this important step forward.

Certainly, you may want the scope of the celebration to match the significance of the milestone. So your celebrations can range from little things, such as taking an afternoon off and going to a movie, to more grand celebrations, such as a weekend at a spa. And, when possible, include in your celebration those people in your support network. It's part of why they're there, and it gives them an opportunity to celebrate their own valuable role.

When I conduct health-change workshops, I ask participants to brainstorm forms of celebration that would be meaningful to them personally, with an eye toward healthful pleasures unrelated to food (just to get them thinking outside the candy box). Here are a few favorites:

- A bubble bath.

- A day of golf.

- A night out with the girls/boys.

- A massage.

- Going dancing.

- Seeing a show.

- Attending a sporting event.

- A special date with a partner or spouse.

- A manicure or pedicure.

- Buying new clothes.

- Going camping.

So go ahead—celebrate your milestones. And remember: These are not "rewards"; you're not a rat, and your well-being is not a maze. When you celebrate your milestones you are, in effect, celebrating *you.*

MIND YOUR CHANGE
What is your next milestone? Think hard. I bet you'll reach one within the next couple of days. Decide today how you will celebrate. Consider one of the celebrations mentioned above, or identify another one that is meaningful to you.

A Little Something Extra
for Yourself

Have you ever driven around with your car's fuel gauge on E? (Who, *you?* No, never, I'm sure!) Perhaps some people get a thrill out of this, but it leaves most of us ill at ease.

On the other hand, isn't there something energizing about driving with a full tank? You can relax a bit; you don't have to keep glancing down at the dashboard. It's just like getting money from the cash machine after you've been walking around penniless for a while. They don't call it "broke" for nothing, you know. When you don't have any money, your energy gets drained like air from a leaky life raft. What if there's an emergency for which you need to travel someplace quickly, or use a pay phone? What would you do? This might not be the biggest stressor in your life, but somewhere in the back of your mind, it's there, weighing you down. Then you go to the ATM, magically withdraw 100 dollars and, next thing you know, you're kicking back at the coffee shop sipping a nonfat caramel macchiato. What the heck, make it a double!

These are examples of a *reserve,* having more than what you immediately need. In coaching, we talk a lot about reserves. "Life coaches" often work with clients on accumulating a financial reserve (not just having more than what you need that day, but having more than what you need in your life). This is one of the many parallels between health and wealth. Wealth represents a reserve of financial resources, and health (in the conventional sense) represents a reserve of physical resources. For example, physical fitness is often defined as the ability to meet both the *ordinary* and the *unusual* challenges of daily life without becoming overly fatigued. You may not agree with this definition, but it illustrates how fitness, an important part of health, is distinctly considered a reserve of physical resources.

Ultimately, all reserves are components of health. To support this concept, you need look no further than the definition of health cited in the introduction to this book: "... a positive concept emphasizing *social and personal resources,* as well as physical capacities."

Following the terrorist attacks of September 11, 2001, I learned an additional lesson about reserves. Throughout the 1990s I lived in California, where residents were continuously reminded by the media to keep emergency kits on hand in the event of a serious earthquake. Despite the virtual certainty of a major quake striking, most Californians didn't heed that advice, and I was no exception.

A couple of weeks before the 9/11 tragedy, my family and I moved from California to upstate New York.

Immediately after the attack, you'll recall, there was tremendous fear about additional acts of mass destruction, chemical warfare, nuclear terrorism, and so forth. Like most Americans, I was fearful. As a father of young children, my mind was full of worst-case scenario images of what the future might hold for my innocent, unsuspecting kids.

After doing some research, especially on the Web site of the American Red Cross, I spent a day assembling an emergency kit. I stashed a few days' worth of food and water, flashlights, batteries, a transistor radio, and all the other things the Red Cross recommended. I attentively chose an appropriate space to store the kit and formulated an emergency action plan with my family.

What I experienced was quite unexpected. While I knew that my supplies might be rendered worthless in the event of a massive attack, immediately upon collecting them I found my fear begin to lift, my sense of helplessness fade. I had taken an important action—really one of the few direct personal actions I could take to address that difficult situation—and in doing so I reclaimed a sense of control over my own life. The emergency kit was, in essence, a safety reserve.

Fortunately, as of this writing, I have not needed to break into that kit in response to a terrorist act. But the part of the country where I now live frequently gets pummeled by snow, hurricane-force winds, and ice storms, which periodically knock out our electricity. So it turns out that I have relied upon those supplies in more than one emergency, and shared them with neighbors, as well.

Reserves exist not only in the form of tangibles, but also in time and space. Most health seekers need to accumulate a reserve of time—that is, to have extra time on their hands—before they can seriously undertake the demands of a health change. Yet this is the type of reserve they resist the most. If you have an ongoing to-do list, then you don't have a reserve of time.

You may believe that every second of your time is supposed to be full, and that having extra time equates with sloth. But being busy isn't virtuous; it's often just another form of escapism. And ultimately, constant busy-ness drains health seekers, depleting their bodies of the energy they need to live life fully, and certainly leaving no fuel for health change.

Furthermore, many health seekers tend to reflexively fill any vacuums in their *physical* environment, guaranteeing that there's no reserve of space. Look at your desk, your filing cabinets, your shelves and drawers, your garage, your property, or even the floor of your home. Is there extra space?

I am reminded of my first stab at gardening. I had acquired, quite by accident, a small cottage garden intensely planted in the backyard by the previous owner of my new home. Just beyond my yard there was a huge lemon tree, probably fifty feet high, with branches spanning thirty feet or so. The tree always had lemons on it, year-round. The lemons were gnarly and inedible, and they weighed down the limbs and continually dropped on my little vegetable patch, where I had planted tomatoes, peppers, and cilantro. Finally, I got tired of the extra work this tree was creating and decided to clear a few of the branches using a long-handled limb pruner.

I cut a few select branches. But as soon as I noticed the glint of sunshine streaming through the cleared overhang, I chose to cut a few more, and then some more. Pretty soon, I had exposed a wide space above my garden, a space that previously had existed only as undiscovered potential. The entire area felt lighter, and I felt lighter being there. I felt connected to the bright sun and the blue sky I had revealed. My garden was transformed. It offered me deep and immediate gratification (and, ultimately, a healthy harvest of ingredients for salsa, too). From this experience, I learned two precious lessons:

1. Extra space facilitates growth. This space often needs to be discovered.

2. When life deals you lemons, don't settle for making lemonade—chop down the lemon tree!

Recall how you felt sometime when you cleaned out a long-cluttered desk drawer or garage, and you'll recognize how energizing a reserve of space can be.

Reserves are an energy wellspring. They offer you readiness in an emergency, they allow you to relax, and they give you room to expand in every dimension of your life. Devise strategies for developing reserves without indulging in excess or depriving others of needed resources. Here are some ideas:

- Develop a plan for financial savings, with professional assistance, if necessary.

- Find new streams of income, such as taking a side job, selling some of your belongings, investing, or acquiring rental property.

- Agree to fewer time-consuming requests. Practice saying no.

- Clear space in your environments. Try a system in which every time you bring an object into your home, you dispose, recycle, or donate something else. An accumulation deficit will lead to a reserve of space.

- Plan appropriately for various types of emergencies.

And don't fall prey to fleeting notions that you may not be entitled to reserves. They are a vital part of the foundation you need in order to make broader changes in your life.

Mind Your Change

There are countless areas in which you can establish reserves, and they all interrelate in one way or another, which means they all bolster the reserve of health and vitality you wish to achieve. I've already mentioned several realms of life that cry out for reserves: finances, safety, time, space, fitness. In which of these can you get started building a reserve today? How about social support, career opportunities, transportation (How will you get to work or school if your car breaks down? Is there another vehicle you can use? Can you ride a bicycle? Do you have access to public transportation?), nourishing environments, and mentors, just to name a few more examples. Only you can determine which realms are most important to you.

CHOOSE WELL

Emma was a high-level manager at a fledgling biotechnology company. In her first coaching session, she told me she felt frustrated by a feeling of falling "out of shape." She had been an active teen and had worked out regularly in her twenties. But four years prior to hiring me as her coach, she had had a baby girl, and now, between work and family, she couldn't find the time to work out. Consequently, she could feel her level of physical fitness diminishing: She got out of breath more easily, often felt fatigued, and was being stalked by our old nemesis, weight gain. This is a common situation, and elsewhere in this book I describe similar cases. Yet each one is unique in terms of what the health seeker learns and how she moves forward.

Emma had told me she was happily married. So, naturally, I asked how her husband fit into all this. Turns out, he was a freelance writer, working on assignments for various national magazines. His work was sporadic, and Emma, according to her own description, was the breadwinner of the family. Yet while her husband was home much of the time, he really hadn't taken on much of the responsibilities of the household. Emma's daughter spent her days in child care, and Emma usually had to hurry home after work to put dinner on the table.

I caution you not to rush to judgment. As a coach, it's not my job to determine what Emma's problem is and how it should be fixed. My job is to help give her the space to clearly identify her own challenges; to guide her to discover the solutions that, someplace inside her, she probably already knows; and to support her as she makes those solutions work.

So what was Emma's challenge? When we dug up the roots, we found that her goal wasn't really fitness. "I'm busy all the time," she told me. "I'm exhausted. I feel like I'm taking care of everybody else at work and at home, and... *[drum roll, please]* I just want to feel like I have some choice in my life."

"Tell me what you mean by that," I said.

"You're right," she replied. It's noteworthy that she said "You're right," because I hadn't said anything to be right about. As clients sometimes do, she was giving me credit for her own excellent insight. Eventually, I would remind her that the brilliance was hers. But back to our story:

"You're right. I do have a choice. I had a choice when I got married, and I knew Aaron was not going to be a breadwinner or a stay-at-home dad. I had a choice when I pursued my career and took my current position. I had a choice when I had a baby. I've had a choice the whole time."

What's my point here, and what does it have to do with health?

My point is that nine times out of ten, you are "at-choice" in your health. I'm not referring to diseases and acute illnesses; sometimes those just happen to you. But when it comes to things like your weight, your eating habits, your fitness level, and your stress—you have created them. You might believe you inherited too many fat cells, or big bones, or muscles that don't work well aerobically. But research has shown that while heredity may affect the upper limits of your fitness level or your tendency to gain weight, most health seekers are more influenced by environmental and behavioral circumstances. If you have no time to exercise, most likely it's because you have chosen to fill your time. If you don't know what foods are healthy, you have chosen not to learn. If you're a stress case because you take care of your kids and your aging parents and hold down two jobs, these also are your choices. This is not to say that you've made the wrong choices. Or the right choices. Just that the choices are yours. You own them. That's what it means to be "at-choice."

If you are unsatisfied with your health, there's no need to malign yourself for creating it the way you have. I don't want you to feel guilty, or remorseful. The lesson here is one of hope: You see, if you have the power to create your health—your weight, your fitness, your stress—then you have the power to *recreate* it, too.

And if you choose *not* to recreate your health, that's fine. But won't you rest easier knowing the decision is yours?

As for Emma, I won't kid you; she had her work cut out for her. Boundaries, over-scheduling, and unmet needs—they were all there, served up on a platter in our very first session. But over time she made remarkable progress, and this was due to her astounding initial insight that she had chosen her life, and she could choose to change it.

MIND YOUR CHANGE
Today, be mindful of every choice you make that influences your physical health negatively or positively. Include things like the foods and beverages you choose to consume, people you have contact with who might have an impact (such as catching a cold from someone or breathing second-hand smoke), extra physical activity you do, media messages to which you expose yourself, use of professional health

services, stress-producing requests you agree to or decline. List these in your journal or in some other convenient place. By the end of a twenty-four-hour period, you will probably list at least fifty. Note how long it will take to manifest the health affects of each choice. Some might make a difference immediately; others might not have significance for many years. As you increase your awareness in this way, you will naturally tend to make choices that are more consistent with the direction in which you want your health, or your life, to go. And you will gain a greater appreciation for the choices available to you that can undo the possible harm of less conscious choices.

The I.F.I.T. Principle

Time was, we health educators and fitness trainers advised people to do aerobic exercise three to five days a week at a certain heart rate for at least twenty minutes. In the 1990s, the U.S. surgeon general and the American College of Sports Medicine (ACSM) standardized a new recommendation: "Accumulate at least thirty minutes of moderate exercise on most, preferably all, days of the week."

What's often overlooked by health seekers, however, is that the new guideline is based on studies of the minimal amount of exercise necessary to prolong life and ward off disease. But I find that, while most people believe that long life and physical health are all well and good, their primary reason for exercising is to manage body weight. I'm not saying this is true of everyone, nor am I making any judgment about it. It's reality, plain and simple.

If you're trying to lose weight, is thirty minutes of moderate exercise enough? Let's look at an example: In accordance with the ACSM guideline, Rhonda walks for thirty minutes five days a week. On average, she walks two miles, which typically will burn about 200 calories. At the end of the week she has exercised away 1000 calories.

How many calories does Rhonda need to burn if she wants to lose weight? Every bit helps, but in one recent study, health seekers who lost at least thirty pounds and kept it off long term burned 2800 calories per week on average through physical activity. Rhonda would have to increase her walking 180 percent to match the profile of a successful weight loser.

Moderate exercise is wonderful, and the guidelines are good. I consistently recommend moderate exercise to clients, and I especially love walking. It keeps you healthier and happier, and it is an appropriate starting point for anyone who can walk. But if you aim to lose substantial weight, be aware of the limitations of moderate exercise. And if you're a walker, plan on about twenty-eight miles over the course of a week (work up to it gradually, though!). Take heed of yet a different set of exercise guidelines, recently issued by the prestigious Institute of Medicine (much to the chagrin of the ACSM), which recommends sixty minutes of moderate exercise every day in order to manage weight.

As I mentioned, the Big Cheeses of the fitness world recommend exercising on *most* days, preferably all. I recommend exercising *nearly every day,* preferably all. It seems like a subtle difference, but it's a difference that can make or break your success. Health seekers who exercise four days a week (this counts as "most" days), or sometimes even five days, are meeting a minimum health requirement but may not be establishing enough continuity in their routine to keep it going.

If you exercise four days a week, then—even if you schedule it into your date book—you're likely to start trading days. *"Okay, I won't work out today, but I'll work out tomorrow, when I wasn't scheduled to."* Problem is, tomorrow comes, and your long-lost cousin Frankie from Buffalo shows up at your door to pay you a visit (or some other unexpected surprise occurs), and next thing you know, the day is done and you haven't exercised. By exercising at least six days a week, you make it part of your life, just like eating and sleeping, and you maintain momentum. I tend to recommend six days rather than seven because I think it's good to rest, and you can do so without losing steam.

If you find that you can maintain momentum exercising five days a week—and many people do, by working out immediately before or after work—fine. But any less than that and there's a sharp drop-off in rates of stick-to-it-ism.

This doesn't mean you have to drive yourself to the limit each day. Perhaps you'll do aerobic exercise on four days and strength training on two days. Or weight training on three days and light stretching on the other three days.

Here's the clincher: What happens on those days when you just don't have the time to exercise? Or when the weather doesn't cooperate? Or when your long-lost cousin visits? Just do *something!* Even if it's just walking around the block. This is one of the best tricks I know for keeping an exercise program going strong.

Let's say it's your scheduled day for a thirty-minute walk in the evening. But you get home from work and realize you have to be at a PTA meeting in half an hour and then get the kids fed and in bed, at which point it will be too late to walk. If you don't have any other options, then go out and walk for five minutes before the meeting, even if it makes you late. Not only will your walk help you relax, but it will maintain your momentum. And momentum is everything. You won't have to deal with the "oh-I-didn't-exercise-like-I-planned-to" blues.

It's that feeling of not doing anything—of failure—that sucks the enthusiasm out of you. On the other hand, it's actually doing something—anything—under difficult circumstances that fortifies your *intent* and will inflate your health confidence to the point where you feel like nothing can stand in your way. Then, nothing *will* stand in your way.

Both the older and newer versions of the exercise guidelines evoke the F.I.T. principle; that is, exercise programs are to be structured around the *frequency, intensity,* and *time* (duration) of activity. Of course, it has been well documented that these guidelines have had little to no effect on the activity habits of Americans. Maybe this is because the guidelines overlooked a key ingredient. When working to maintain a fitness program over the long haul (or for that matter, integrating any new health habit into your life), it's not quantity or quality, but your *intent* that matters most.

I present to you . . . the I.F.I.T. principle: *intent,* frequency, intensity, and time.

Have a great workout!

MIND YOUR CHANGE
Your intent to exercise regularly can be supported by staying motivated, committing to consistency, and giving high priority to your fitness. This handbook is chock-full of practical tips for doing just that. For starters, bone up on the chapters "Power-Up Health Confidence," "How to Make Health Fit," and "From Resolutions to Real Solutions."

GET ON THE BALL:
THE BENEFITS OF MIND/BODY EXERCISE

TEN years ago, while employed as general manager of a popular dance exercise company, I played a lead role in popularizing Pilates. My company helped coax this elaborate system of movements out of the dance world, where it was a well-kept secret for many decades, and successfully promoted it to the broader population of fitness enthusiasts. So it is with a sense of irony that I now witness the explosion of Pilates exercise, which is featured in seemingly endless television infomercials and in numerous best-selling books and videos. While I find most hot fitness trends to be little more than exercises in futility, I continue to endorse Pilates. In fact, I strongly believe that mind/body exercise, such as Pilates, should be a part of every health seeker's workout routine. It's relaxing, energizing, and empowering, and by enhancing body awareness it facilitates other health changes you may want to make.

Of course, your choices for mind/body exercise go well beyond Pilates. Yoga and tai chi, for example, offer profound mind/body experiences. In fact, any system of movement that requires you to focus 100 percent of your attention on purposeful, flowing movements, coordinated with attentive breathing, qualifies as mind/body exercise.

Exercising on inflatable workout balls is a popular trend that also happens to be worthwhile. Performing controlled, precise movements on an unstable surface activates important muscles that otherwise tend to go untrained. I especially recommend ball workout routines that incorporate Pilates and yoga techniques, as opposed to using the ball simply as an accessory in a standard strength training or aerobic workout. These allow you to fully explore the ball as a tool for mind/body integration, rather than utilizing it as just another piece of gym equipment.

All of these mind/body exercises build "core strength," training the deep muscles in and around the abdomen and back. Not only is core strength key to maintaining good posture and preventing back injury, but it is the foundation of your overall body strength. Even elite strength-oriented athletes like football players emphasize core strength in their training regimens.

Just as importantly, mind/body exercise promotes *mindfulness*. As you bring your attention to the movement you are doing, there is little opportunity for other distractions—such as the proverbial preoccupations with past events and future planning—to elbow their way in there. During mind/body exercise, you will be truly present, and you will carry that presence beyond the workout and feel refreshed and invigorated. As such, mind/body exercise is a particularly helpful practice for health seekers who wish to cultivate mindfulness but who aren't naturally inclined to slow down or still their bodies. (Mindfulness is discussed in much greater detail in the next section.)

If the concept of mind/body exercise is new to you, you can get a sense of its potential with this analogy: Imagine a powerful telescope that enables you to see worlds that would otherwise not be visible to you. This instrument relies on two well-crafted lenses that are precisely adjusted to bring your field of view into perfect focus. Misalign these lenses, and everything gets blurry. Realign them, and the worlds you are observing become clearer.

You are like this instrument. Your body and your mind are lenses. You perceive your world one way with your body and another way with your mind. And when your body and your mind are perfectly attuned to each other—which is exactly what occurs as a result of mind/body exercise—your perception of the world becomes exponentially more acute and more expansive, just like that view through a fine telescope.

So take a breather from the results-oriented intensity of pedestrian exercise, and spend time enjoying the integration of your mind and your body. After all, that's what they're there for.

MIND YOUR CHANGE
Make a commitment today to try some form of mind/body exercise. Rent a yoga video at the library or video store, make an appointment for a complimentary session if there's a Pilates studio near you, or sign up for a tai chi class through your local recreation department. Commit to test these waters unencumbered by preconceived notions.

Part II
Trim Down

Mindfulness:
The Secret to Health Change?

If there is a secret to successful health change, it lies in mindfulness—full awareness of the present moment. Regular mindfulness practice—focusing your attention, without judgment, to what is right here, right now—will reduce or eliminate the difficulties you may encounter as you change your health behavior or any other aspect of your life. For example, it will:

- Increase your awareness of what triggers unhealthy behaviors.

- Help you keep unhealthy cravings at bay.

- Elevate your sense of well-being—free from stresses about the future or the past—so you will intuitively take better care of yourself, rather than trying to force it with willpower.

- Enable you to cope with relapses without guilt, and with overall equanimity.

- Liberate you from comparing yourself to other people.

- Provide you with a healthful means to deal with anger, anxiety, or feelings of low self-worth, so these common and deep-seated emotions don't undermine you.

- Instruct you in how to "let go" of circumstances that keep you stuck.

That's the big picture. But mindfulness can help you gain immediate returns in your everyday life, as well.

- Practice mindfulness while eating—paying complete and quiet attention to the present moment and being aware of all perceptions related to eating—and you will find that you can naturally choose healthy foods, eat moderate portions, and "tune in" to your sense of satiation.

- Practice mindfulness while exercising, and you can eliminate boredom and shed those internal voices that generate reasons not to exercise.

- Practice mindfulness at work and when interacting with coworkers, and you will reduce your work-related stress.

If you are trying to change an unhealthy habit, your success will surely be facilitated by mindfulness. Let's say that every night you watch television, and whenever you settle in front of the TV you break out a bag of potato chips. This is so customary for you that night after night you find yourself sitting there munching, without having any recollection of putting yourself in that situation, and without ever even deciding *"This is how I'll spend my evening."* You want to change this behavior, but how *can* you if you're not even present when it occurs? With mindfulness in your life, you will be present. You will become aware of the impulse to turn the TV on, or to grab the chips, and you will be able to let go of that impulse without having to bear down on it.

Mindfulness is unfettered by memories of the past, plans for the future, judgments, random thoughts, and overpowering feelings. To practice mindfulness, bring your mind to the present moment. When it strays, bring it back, over and over again. Observation of your breath is one of the best tools for doing this; let it show you the way. Your breath is always there with you, and it acts to unify your body and your mind. Bring your attention to your breath, noticing the air as it enters your nostrils and wends its way down to your lungs. And then, upon exhalation, notice it return to the external world. Feel your chest or abdomen rising and falling as you breathe. Relax, as if you were breathing relaxation directly into the muscles of your body and into your mind. This does not require much effort, and you can be mindful of your breathing as well as anything else you're doing, be it working, washing dishes, walking, or what have you. In fact, as you return your attention to your breath, in the present moment, over and over again, you will indeed be mindful of whatever it is you are doing and wherever you are in that moment. Try it right now, as you read: Breathe in and notice your breath. Breathe out and notice your breath.

Pay attention. Inevitably, thoughts, memories, plans, and powerful emotions will enter your mind. This is as it should be. Do not strive to eliminate mental activity. After all, your mind's job description includes thinking, planning, feeling, remembering, and miscellaneous duties as assigned. So don't turn this into a battle by trying to eliminate these things. And don't suppress them. Simply observe them, and let them go.

Newcomers to the practice of mindfulness often assume that they should suppress their thoughts. But nothing could be further from the truth. Letting go of thoughts via the practice of mindfulness is the exact opposite of suppression. As long as you try to suppress thoughts, and the feelings that may lie at their roots, they will continue to provoke upheaval, seeking to express themselves in some way. Suppressed thoughts, often unknown to us, can lead to health problems, both mental and physical.

How do you let go of thoughts? One of the best techniques is to label them. Let's say you're practicing mindfulness and you start thinking about an argument you had with your spouse that morning. You observe the thought and gently say to yourself, *"Remembering,"* and return to your breath. Or you may choose to say, *"Anger,"* if that's what you're feeling. By labeling your distractions, you purposefully acknowledge rather than suppress them. When you acknowledge them, you release them. But when you suppress them, you merely perpetuate their presence.

If you are practicing mindfulness and you encounter particularly difficult emotions, acknowledge them in the friendliest of ways, as if you are greeting an old friend. *"Ah, anger, nice to see you again,"* or *"My old friend, self-criticism."* No need to use all these words to label these visitors, but you can greet them with this kind of demeanor. This is especially effective for health seekers who meet resistance to their mindfulness, to their health change, or to their lives. Remember, resistance is that tug-of-war you set up within yourself, the one you can never win. Greet your greatest challenges as your friends rather than as your adversaries, and your resistance will recede. Any intentions you have about overcoming, beating, or surmounting will help neither your mindfulness nor your health change. If you see yourself, even a facet of yourself, as something to be overcome, then you are viewing yourself as the enemy. This may be part of the problem. Certainly it is not part of the solution.

When practicing mindfulness, don't allow judgment to distract you. You may be one of those people who keeps a judge's scorecard in your mind. At times, you assign comparative scores: *"This is a pretty good book, but not as good as the last one I read. I wonder if I'll be able to relate to the next chapter as well as I relate to this chapter..."* Often, the judgments are about yourself: *"Why can't I be as organized as my neighbor?"* And when you practice mindfulness, you may even find that your judging mind is issuing a running commentary about the quality of your mindfulness: *"Breathe in. Breathe out. Breathe in... Gosh, my breathing is fast. I wonder if it's because of that cup of coffee I drank? Or is it always like that and I usually don't... Darn! I was practicing mindfulness and now I'm lost in thought. Why can't I do this better? I must be doing it wrong."*

When you notice yourself drifting like this, just say to yourself, *"Judging,"* and return to your breath without further judgment. Judging your mindfulness is just another means of avoiding the present.

There's a school of coaches that's fond of saying "The present is perfect." What a nice idea. But even "is perfect" represents a judgment, albeit a positive judgment. In your practice of mindfulness, positive judgment is not much better than negative judgment. Embrace equanimity. The present is...the present. If you judge the present to be perfect in this moment, you are just as likely to judge the present as unsatisfactory in some other moment. By practicing mindfulness without judgment, you can let go of this habit of judging and enjoy the experience of the present moment without bothering about whether it's a good moment or a bad moment.

Mindfulness can be practiced at any time, no matter what you're doing. To strengthen your practice of mindfulness, however, I recommend that you practice for at least a few minutes every day in a controlled environment. For example, if you have a room in your home where you can dim the lights and lie down on the floor, flat on your back, with peace and quiet for a few minutes, then try it. Lie there, with your eyes open or closed—whatever's comfortable for you—and practice mindfulness, simply observing your breath and paying attention to the present moment. This is not a trance-like condition. It's just the opposite—a time of heightened awareness. Be aware of sounds, of the feeling of the floor supporting you, and of the position of your body. These are all there in the present moment.

If it helps, you also can practice with music. Focus your attention on the beautiful sound as you observe your breath coming in and going out. Or, if you like to walk, practice mindful walking—watching your breath as you feel each foot taking a step and making contact with the ground.

Another excellent way to practice mindfulness is to eat mindfully. You can start with a simple healthy snack, such as a box of raisins or a piece of fruit. Commit 100 percent of your attention to the act of eating. Be fully aware of opening the box of raisins or slicing the fruit. Be aware of your body as you bring the snack to your mouth. What are the physical sensations you are experiencing? Put the food in your mouth, and chew each bite at least thirty times. Be aware of the tastes, textures, and smells, and of the feelings that are evoked. Feel the food go down as you swallow it. All the while, anchor yourself in the present with your breath. Take a few moments between bites to relax and simply be mindful of your breath and of the sensations of having eaten. Then mindfully take the next bite. Mindful eating is a powerful experience. Anyone trying to alter eating habits must try it. After all, you cannot change your habits unless you are present when they occur. Beyond that, though, mindful eating is a fundamental mindfulness practice for anyone. If you find you enjoy it, try eating at least one meal a week in quiet mindfulness.

These types of mindful practices under controlled circumstances, akin to meditation, are like practicing a musical scale on an instrument, learning the structure so well that you will be able to improvise readily and naturally. Practice mindfulness in a controlled setting, and with increasing spontaneity you will return to the present moment throughout your day-to-day life, and your experience of the present will deepen.

Don't be discouraged if you find that the more you practice, the less mindful you feel. It may seem like your mind is jumping around more than ever. This is commonly called "the monkey mind," based on the image of chattering monkeys leaping from tree to tree, just as the mind jumps from thought to thought. One mindfulness teacher I used to study with compared our practice to cleaning a room. "The more you clean that room," he said, "the more dirt you see. As you scrub the floors, scratches become more visible. Clean the windows, and you chase after streaks. Start dusting, and you notice the layer of grit on the baseboard, which you never noticed before. So it is with your mind. As you become more and more mindful, you become more and more aware of your distraction. It seems as if your monkey mind is wilder than ever. But in reality, you are more aware of it than you ever were. And that's the first step to taming the monkey."

When your practice of mindfulness deepens, after much time and experience, you may encounter discomforting emotions or thoughts. This can be challenging at first. It may be that you have avoided these emotions, because they are simply too painful to confront and you haven't been equipped to do so. But remember the distinction between *acknowledging and releasing* difficult emotions versus *suppressing and perpetuating* them. Consider how this may apply to you. If you've been trying for a long time to lose weight, eat better, get fit, or reduce stress and have only met with frustrating results, recognize that perhaps your efforts are being sabotaged by some unidentified internal dynamic. Through this kind of more advanced practice of mindfulness, you can cut a swath through the various mental weeds that have germinated under the guise of protecting you, and you can see what's really holding you back. You may wish to seek the help of a coach, therapist, or spiritual instructor as you delve this deeply into your practice of mindfulness.

But mindfulness is not all about confronting the unpleasant. On the contrary. As you practice mindfulness, you will find that there is joy in the present moment—always. Even when life circumstances can seem quite grim, through mindfulness you will find that it is your *reactions* to circumstances that generate your difficulty. But joy is your natural state, and you can visit this state through mindfulness. You can be steady in the storm.

Not only will your practice of mindfulness improve *your* life, but it will improve the lives of those around you. As a coach, I have received considerable training in listening skills, and I believe that I have a natural propensity for good listening. And

I can tell you this: Good listening *is* the practice of mindfulness. When a friend speaks and you give her your undivided attention—without judging what she says and without formulating your response, but simply listening in the present moment—you are practicing mindfulness. Similarly, when you speak skillfully to your friend—taking care that your words accurately express what you wish but are not hurtful or manipulative—again, you are practicing mindfulness.

So much stress, in families, in the workplace—everywhere in society—is related to faulty communication and difficult interaction. Imagine how much better off we all would be if we maintained mindfulness, as I have described it, in our exchanges with each other.

And incidentally, while I do extol the benefits of mindfulness as they relate to health change, I don't believe that change is impossible in the absence of a dedicated mindfulness practice. But if you have tried the eight-week plans, the six-step programs, the formulas, the treatments, the pills, the shakes, the healers, the crystals, and everything else under the sun, I urge you ultimately to rest your attention on mindfulness. You have nothing to lose but your distractions.

MIND YOUR CHANGE
Many unhealthy habits are associated with specific triggers. Smokers, for example, may be more likely to light up when they're drinking a cup of coffee or when they're in a bar. Many health seekers indulge in unhealthful snacks when they watch TV. Some grab a candy bar from the vending machine

at work when they're up against a deadline. But you also can use triggers to your advantage by establishing a system for triggering a healthy behavior, such as mindfulness. Decide on a cue that you know you will encounter several times today to serve as a trigger for mindfulness. It can be the sound of your phone ringing, an incoming e-mail alert, or observing something in nature, such as a bird—whatever works best for you. Then, throughout your day, when your trigger appears, bring your attention to your breath and the present moment, and hold your attention there.

If you wish to find out more about mindfulness, or to explore additional techniques for cultivating it in your everyday life, many useful books are available. I especially recommend the works of Thich Nhat Hanh, from whom I have adopted many of the mindfulness techniques described in this chapter. Check the "Recommended Reading" section at the back of this book for more information.

GET UNSTUCK BY LETTING GO

IF you're like most people, then at times you have probably felt "stuck" in your pursuit of better health. I find that when health seekers feel stuck, more often than not they are actually *holding on*—unwilling, unprepared, or unable to let go.

To improve your health, there is no end to the list of things you may need to let go of. Here are some of the most common:

- *Old goals.* If you've had the same goal for, say, several years, with no signs of progress, it's probably time to let it go. Then you'll have room for new goals. If you can let go of your weight-loss goal, maybe you'll adopt a new, previously unimaginable goal. Maybe your goal will be to hike from Maine to Georgia. And you might just shed a few pounds in the process.

- *Perfectionism/Absolutism.* "*I'm going to stop eating sugar in every form!*" Really? Sounds like a set-up for failure. If you can let go of that idea, maybe you can adopt a more reasonable goal, such as indulging in sweets no more than once a week.

- *Shoulds.* Countless times, I've seen health seekers fixate on the type of exercise they think they *should* be doing (such as using whatever piece of home exercise equipment they have), and they never do it. They cling to their *shoulds* and never stop to consider what their *wants* are. This is part of eliminating resistance: Stop wasting time with your *shoulds* and embrace your *wants.* Unless required for medical reasons, you're not likely to do a *should* for the rest of your life (regardless of whether that *should* is riding your stationary bike, taking a vitamin daily, meditating, balancing your checkbook, or whatever). It's easy to commit to a *want*.

- *Other people's goals for you.* Oh, there's no shortage of them. Your husband wants you to be thinner; your mother thinks you should eat more vegetables; Madison Avenue wants you to stay young forever. You can't even hear your own goals in your mind until you can get everyone else's to stop clanging around in there.

- *Fear.* Health seekers fabricate all sorts of reasons to avoid taking actions that scare them. Often what they fear is failure. With more clinical types of health changes, such as doing regular breast self-exams, they fear a catastrophic finding. Letting go of fear is hard, but you can do it.

- *Other people's doings.* Comparing yourself to others is a losing proposition. Don't concern yourself with how your neighbor is doing with her weight loss, her fitness, her stress, or her life. They're hers, not yours.

In the opening words to the introduction of this book, I depicted willpower as a bulldog that ensnares you and won't let go. But at this point, I invite you to reconsider that image. Is it the willpower that won't let go? Or are *you* unwilling to let go of your faith in willpower (regardless of its dismal track record)?

Letting go pervades every aspect of your life. For example, when you forgive someone for something he has done to hurt you, you let go of your resentment. This perfectly exemplifies the healing power of letting go. As you let go of your resentment, not only do you give the other person a chance to feel better, but you unburden yourself from the harmful effects of holding a grudge. As long as resentment is allowed to fester inside you, it will undermine you emotionally and physically.

Charitable giving is another example of letting go. It represents letting go of your attachment to wealth or material things; or, in the case of volunteering, your sense that your time is, indeed, your own.

Even disposing of or recycling possessions is an important act of letting go. You probably know some people who are pack rats, saving everything that crosses their path, cluttering up their closets, drawers, basements, garages, attics, and file cabinets with stuff they will never use or need. Perhaps this describes you. Usually, you'll find that this inability to let go of "stuff" goes hand in hand with an inability to let go of intangibles: old goals and beliefs, past relationships, previous positions in society or in the workplace, and, generally, the "good old days."

Any time you let go, whether it be forgiveness, charity, or simply letting go of beliefs about your health change, you make it easier to let go the next time. Letting go is like a semicharged flow of energy through your life. And whenever you intentionally let go of something—*anything*—it adds to that charge, allowing the energy to flow more strongly.

Letting go is of great importance—*ultimate* importance, far beyond even your health change. After all, the day will come in your life—it will be the last day—when you must let go of everything, including everything that is dear to you: your family, everything you have ever known, your very self. You'll have to let go of nothing less than life itself. I've heard it said that the difference between a "good death" and a "difficult death" depends on how readily the departing person can let go. So isn't now a good time to tend to this skill? It does require practice, and practicing doesn't hurt one bit. Just the opposite—practice letting go and you will add that charge of energy in your life. Everything will become lighter and come more easily to you. Even your health change.

This is part of why mindfulness is so important. Mindfulness *is* an act of letting go, in its most fundamental form. Each time you return to your breath—letting go of thinking, planning, remembering, judging, comparing, and so forth—you are practicing letting go. As you do so, you gather the strength to let go of the things to which you are most attached—the things that keep you the most stuck.

When you first set your intention on letting go, resistance will arise. Resistance is generally driven by fear. *"What's there, after I let go?"*

Imagine yourself stranded at sea, clinging to a life preserver. You may feel stuck. But really, you are not letting go. It would be stupid to let go, wouldn't it?

Maybe not. It wouldn't be stupid to let go if there's something else, something solid and grounded, for you to move toward. For this reason, when I work with health seekers on letting go of goals and beliefs that keep them stuck, we first work to discover their possibility, just as I mentioned in the first chapter of this book. From this possibility is born the vision they will move toward once they have let go.

Discovering your possibility alleviates your fear of letting go. And after you have practiced for a while and have grown increasingly comfortable with letting go, you may get to the point where you can even let go of your possibility. Then, the depth of your unlimited potential can truly be explored.

Now, what do *you* need to let go of?

MIND YOUR CHANGE

Watch the video *Cast Away* starring Tom Hanks, even if you've seen it before. Note that it is not about a guy stuck on an island. It is a profound and stirring story about letting go. It's about casting away.

STAVING OFF BOREDOM

WHEN I coach a client on eating healthier, exercising, losing weight, or managing stress, I can anticipate when boredom will strike, usually a couple of weeks before it actually does. The client's voice loses its charge when she talks about her modified lifestyle. Newly acquired health habits almost imperceptibly begin to move down her priority list. And her possibility fades from the forefront of our coaching sessions, like a dropped flashlight sinking into a murky pond.

Generally, boredom is preceded by a slowing in the rate of the client's progress. Think about it: If you wanted to lose thirty pounds via healthy eating and exercise, and you were losing a pound a day, you'd easily reach your goal without getting bored. But if you lost five pounds the first week, and then it took you twelve weeks to lose the next two pounds, you'd start running out of enthusiasm.

When I detect the early signs of boredom, I encourage clients to return to their "beginner's mind," a term popularized by Shunryu Suzuki in his classic book *Zen Mind, Beginner's Mind*. Of course, there are many well-known strategies for coping with boredom: adding variety to your routine, setting new goals, and so forth. But with beginner's mind, I offer you a new arrow for your quiver, an arrow that is especially likely to hit its target.

How does beginner's mind work in this context? Here's an example: If I'm coaching a walker who's starting to find walking tedious, I would encourage her to tap in to the feelings she experienced during our very first coaching call. "Take yourself back to that place," I might say. "Relive the excitement you had then ... the hope. Next time you lace up your walking shoes and go for your walk, pretend it's your first-ever fitness walk. Take note of the elevated heart rate and the light beads of perspiration as if you weren't expecting them. Be mindful even of the swelling that occurs in your fingers, with the curiosity you experienced that very first time. Resurrect the enthusiasm of a fresh start."

And since most of my clients keep journals, I would encourage this client to reread those entries from the time when she first started walking, or even just before that, when she was first considering it. This would help her rediscover her original motivation, her energy, and her possibility.

Your beginner's mind is a gift you give to yourself. All you need to do is unwrap it. For staving off boredom, it is consistently effective. And you may find it offers great rewards beyond that.

Many people say, "Live each day as if it were your last." Successful health seekers say, "Live each day as if it were your first!"

MIND YOUR CHANGE

What aspect of your life is getting boring to you? Your health pursuits? Your job? School? A relationship? Take yourself back to your very first day and ask yourself: What was the best thing about starting? What were your hopes and dreams on that day? How did you feel, and what were your physical sensations?

Unwrap your beginner's mind.

How to Make Health Fit

HEALTH seekers sabotage themselves when they take on the intense work of health improvement without creating space for it to fit into their otherwise busy lives. Yet in working with coaching clients who've been trying to make some kind of health change, I've noticed that many have been stuck for a long time for exactly that reason: Between the responsibilities of their careers, their families, and everyday life, they have little left for themselves.

Roger was a classic example. A sales director for a large manufacturing firm in Seattle, married with two teenagers, Roger first came to me as a client when he was in his early forties. Roger's sales job kept him running (figuratively speaking). He was on the road much of the time, both locally and nationwide. His department was held to ambitious quotas. Roger had input into these quotas, but he admitted that due to his driven personality, he liked them set high enough to keep him from resting on his laurels. He aspired eventually to have a position as vice president in the company, and he was taking two classes per semester at the local university as he worked toward a master's degree in business administration.

Roger's wellness goal at the time was to improve every aspect of his health. He wanted to return to the type of exercise program he had maintained in his early twenties, before he had kids, which included regular strength training with weights and jogging three to five miles five days a week. He wanted to lose the twenty pounds he had gained over the past fifteen years. He also recognized that as a result of working about fifty-five hours a week while trying to devote appropriate time to his family, he was running himself ragged, and he wanted to reduce his stress. His hectic lifestyle led to other unhealthful habits, such as relying on fast food for lunch. He was aware that this was harmful and wanted to eat healthier, maybe even cut out red meat altogether. Roger also knew that his fluid intake of almost exclusively diet cola was less than ideal, and he wanted to start drinking at least eight glasses of water a day.

Roger wanted, Roger wanted. Roger wanted a lot. Perhaps you know a Roger. Perhaps you *are* a Roger. Either way, you might be amazed at how many Rogers there are in the world. I would say that more than half of the clients who contact me are highly driven health seekers whose lives could be described as nothing less than frenetic. Roger was what we used to call a Type A personality—what lots of coaches call "running on adrenaline." It's especially common among sales professionals, but I see it in every walk of life—from doctors, to artists, to homemakers. Often when these health seekers turn their attention to health, they do it with the same turbo-drive with which they attack every other aspect of their lives. They take on drastic changes that last a few weeks, and then—bang!—not only do they crash and end up right back where they started, but sometimes they slip back even further than that.

After talking to Roger for just a few minutes—a conversation throughout which his cell phone was ringing, his pager was chirping, and his e-mail notification was pinging—I could tell that he was remarkably self-aware, and that he had managed to look at his lifestyle objectively. What he saw was that not only was he killing himself with stress, unhealthy eating, a sedentary lifestyle, and more stress, but he exemplified the classic gerbil-in-the-wheel syndrome: the faster he ran, the further away his goals seemed to be. Work was getting harder. His family life was filled with tension. His money wasn't buying him happiness.

Roger needed to take care of himself. But even if he knew exactly what to do for exercise, how to integrate healthy eating into his life, and how to practice stress management, when in the world would he do it all?

Roger's natural inclination was to try to shoehorn these things into his current lifestyle. He was going to wake up earlier to go to the gym every single day. He was going to cook big batches of healthy foods on Sundays and take leftovers to work for lunch. He had bought three books about raising teenagers, and while he couldn't find time to read them, in skimming them he noticed that each book recommended family meetings, so he was going to start that, too.

I kid you not. Roger really planned on doing all these things.

This is where I, as a coach, really earn my keep.

I can tell you flat-out, unequivocally, and without reservation that Roger needed to slow down before he did anything else. He was unable to manage the things he was already doing—so how could he take on more? He needed to have time for himself, to simplify his life. To accomplish this, he was going to have to let go of existing plans and projects. This is the single most important action to be taken by most health seekers who want to make successful, lasting health change—even if they're not Type A's (after all, Roger is an extreme example). And yet it's the action they resist most strongly. Letting go of busy-ness is hard, but like any other act of letting go, it is possible. And it can be accomplished with decreased resistance as you continue to hone your letting-go skill through the practice of mindfulness.

In one of our early sessions, before Roger embarked on any big exercise or nutritional programs, I made this simple request of him: "Roger, this week I would like you to drink eight glasses of water every day. I want you to drink each glass over the course of no less than five minutes, and I don't want you to do anything else while you're drinking. Turn your pager, cell phone, and e-mail program off, and simply sit, quietly, as you drink."

I had a few reasons for making this request. Part of my job is to encourage people to think big—to stretch their goals. With some health seekers, thinking big may mean striving for more. But with many, Roger included, thinking big means doing less. Also, I knew Roger was eager to get started, perhaps secretly hoping I'd give him a two-hour-a-day exercise program. And I did want him to get a sense of accomplishment. He needed to feel like he was moving forward and to learn what it felt like to make a change in his life.

At our next session, however, Roger reported that he was unable to meet that week's goal. He didn't have time to sit down and drink water. "How much time do you think you'll need to commit to exercise, healthy meal preparation, and stress reduction, if you want to meet your goals, Roger?" I asked.

"I see where you're going," he said. "If I don't have time to drink a few glasses of water, how will I have time to do all those other things?"

In the ensuing months, as I helped Roger identify what he really wanted and what was important to him, he made dramatic modifications to his lifestyle. He got his sales quotas adjusted downward, he took breaks in his day for relaxing and for mindful water drinking, and he dropped out of business school.

As you read this, you may be shocked. Dropped out of business school?! *"Bob, you ruined this guy's life!"* you may think. Of course, there was a lot of coaching around that decision. But ultimately, the decision was all Roger's. In an e-mail he sent to me some time later, here's what he had to say about it:

"I can't believe how much my life has changed. For the first time in my adult life, I feel in control. I don't bring my job home with me, and finally I have time for myself. I even have come to see my time with my family as time for myself, because being with them is one of the greatest pleasures I have. At first I felt guilty about leaving biz school, I felt like I was giving up. But now I see that that was the best decision I ever made. Thinking back, I realize that I hated business school, and that I can probably get the advance in my career that I want even without the MBA. Underneath it all, I think I wanted to quit the MBA program from the first day I started, and what really helped was having someone tell me that that decision was okay. My job is going well, and while the family still has its struggles, we are working with a counselor and have a renewed sense of hopefulness. I am working out regularly, lifting weights and taking long walks, and I feel vibrant and alive. The road I was on, I suspect, was going to give me a heart attack. Slowing down saved my life."

"P.S.," he wrote, "I still drink my water. It's very refreshing."

We live in a society that is confused about work and busyness. We pay lip service to the importance of slowing down and taking time for ourselves, yet something keeps us running in circles. If we do slow down and create free time, we are wracked with guilt. So many of my clients complain about how busy they are, yet in their voices I hear an element of braggadocio in their complaining. Frenzy is the condition health seekers love to hate. When I suggest that clients schedule into their week a few hours to do nothing—scheduling unscheduled time—they react with confusion, resistance, and sometimes even a bit of resentment. They believe unscheduled time is decadent. Yet inevitably it is out of this quiet time that their possibilities become reality. And to think that you can achieve any real sense of well-being while leading a frenetic life—or that you can cram new healthy behaviors into a life that already is overpacked to bursting—is just plain wrong.

Have you ever done that exercise where you draw a circle and divide it like a pie chart, based on how much of your total time you spend doing different things? Often it's called "The Wheel of Life." Most people look at their wheel and are struck by the imbalances. For instance, the career slice may be more than half the wheel, while the things they love doing the most, whether it's family time, gardening, or perhaps reading, are a barely visible sliver.

Changing your health takes a lot of energy, and usually a lot of time, as well. Cooking healthier meals, working out, doing relaxation exercises, meeting with support groups—it all consumes time. Staying motivated requires energy. Even giving something up—such as sugary snacks or caffeine—can be exhausting, both physically and mentally. So, can you cram these things into your wheel of life? No. You need to create space.

Creating space won't require sacrifice. A lack of balance in your life may have led to unhealthy habits in the first place. Rebalancing, by putting more time aside for yourself, is likely to be a welcome relief.

I recommend five strategies to help you create space in your life. I've had clients who have taken these steps as a leap of faith and been startled by the payoff. The strategies are:

1. *Deflect.* At the outset of your health change, don't take on new projects, chores, or tasks.

2. *Drop.* You know all of those tasks you do that take up all your time? Don't do them all. Look hard at these things and ask yourself, "Why?" What are your priorities, and where does your well-being fit in? Drop what you don't need to do.

3. *Distill.* Simplify your life. Check your e-mail and voicemail no more than twice a day. Sell, donate, or dispose of stuff you don't need. If you bring a new possession into your home, take something else out.

4. *Delegate.* If you can afford to pay someone else to clean your home, or mow your lawn, or wash your dog, do it. And work with your fellow householders to make sure they're carrying their weight with housework.

5. *De-Should.* Your energy is drained not just by all the things you do, but by everything you think you should be doing but aren't. Examples: getting more education, upgrading the house, writing a book, throwing a party.

At first, you'll resist these kinds of measures. They may seem impossible, and they're nothing like the health tips the mainstream media feeds you. But when you modify a health habit, you're making a monumental shift you want to stick with for the rest of your life. So isn't it natural that you need to jolt your life a bit to do it?

In a previous chapter, "A Little Something Extra for Yourself," I wrote about the value of building reserves of time and physical space. Building reserves and creating space are not the same thing, though they are part of the same spectrum and the distinction is subtle. When you build reserves, you go beyond creating space—you *accrue* space. But when you create space, you *eliminate the deficits* in your time, space, and other areas of life.

The bottom line is, you must create space before you can build reserves.

Mind Your Change

Make a Not-To-Do List. Include anything you've thought you should do, but which really isn't as important as your health change. Cross items off your list as you become confident that you have let go of them.

TURN OFF YOUR TV

TELEVISION is the vortex in which health seekers' most earnest efforts often veer off course.

Research has convincingly shown that TV is hazardous to your health. For example, a study of more than 4,000 men and women, ages twenty-three to thirty-five years, found that lengthy TV viewing is associated with obesity, physical inactivity, depression, hostility, alcoholism, and smoking. Another study of more than 50,000 women showed that for every two hours of TV watched per day, there is a 23 percent increase in obesity and a 14 percent increase in risk of diabetes. And perhaps most relevant to health seekers: TV watching was closely tied to relapse in a study of otherwise successful weight loss program participants.

These statistics aren't surprising. TV is a sedentary pastime, and no one disputes the correlation between inactivity and obesity. Recently, however, researchers found that, as a sedentary activity, TV watching is in a class all its own. It slows your metabolism even further than other restful activities, such as reading or just sitting around. Think about it: You burn more calories sitting in a chair and looking at the birds outside your window than you do watching your favorite sitcom.

The damaging effects of TV, however, are not limited to those resulting from its position as the cornerstone of sedentary life. Television programming aggressively promotes unhealthy products and slyly portrays people consuming those products without any ill effects, and it perpetuates harmful myths about what healthy bodies look like.

Health seekers often tell me they are drawn to TV after a stressful day at work. In such cases, I advise them to pay attention to how they feel when they finally turn the TV off. Calm? Rejuvenated? No. Generally, their stress persists. And though they feel drained, they frequently have difficulty sleeping. When they trade at least some of that TV time, however, for exercise, creative arts, social interaction, journaling, or even volunteer work, they find they have more energy throughout the day, and they tend to enjoy more peaceful sleep through the night.

In other cases I've known, health seekers who aspire to adopt wholesome eating habits meet great success during the day, but when prime time arrives, they turn on the TV and binge on junk food. This can be complicated. You might think that the TV triggers their binge, but I find that, in some cases, these health seekers have not dealt effectively with their junk food cravings, and they use "the tube" to drown out the negative feelings they associate with indulgence. In either case, the practice of mindfulness—paying close attention to their behavior, their environment, and their feelings in the present moment—serves as a current on which they can sail out of the TV vortex.

I don't necessarily advise health seekers to forego TV entirely (I don't advise against it either). My clients have found it helpful to conduct a TV "fast" for a period of time, ranging from one weekend to one month. This helps them acclimate to life without TV. Then, if they choose to reintroduce TV into their lives, they naturally do so with greater consciousness and discernment. They watch only the programs they want to watch, rather than sitting there waiting for something good to come on. They control the TV, rather than letting it control them. You can do the same.

MIND YOUR CHANGE

Conduct a TV fast for a period of one week. During this time:

- Move your television to a less prominent location.

- Avoid the TV schedule in the newspaper.

- Plan positive activities for some of those times when you ordinarily watch TV.

- Don't replace your TV time with other media, such as movies or internet.

If you need support, contact the TV-Turnoff Network in Washington, D.C. They can provide you with loads of ideas and resources.

COPING WITH CRAVINGS

A$_T$ some point during the change process, health seekers inevitably encounter cravings. If you're trying to reduce your intake of fat, sugar, or salt, you will at times crave those taste sensations. Quitting cigarettes? Of course you'll crave a smoke. The same goes for caffeine. If you're starting an exercise program, at the end of the day when you're leaving work and scheduled to head over to the gym, you just might experience a craving to do something else: go home and watch TV, work a little more, grab a pizza.

Intrinsically linked to craving is feeling deprived. Health seekers tend to crave whatever they feel they are being deprived of. Deep down, they believe that if they satisfy their craving, the uncomfortable feeling of deprivation will go away. But unfortunately, it doesn't always work that way.

When faced with a craving, you have three options:

1. You can try to suppress the craving.

2. You can submit to the craving.

3. You can choose to neither suppress nor submit to the craving.

The third possibility is your best option to support the long-term success of your health improvement.

Coping with cravings is a natural extension of the skills you have acquired or can acquire via the practice of mindfulness (raw attention to the present moment). When you practice mindfulness, your mind is like a calm sea. And then a huge wave comes along in the form of a distraction. Can you stop a wave? Will you allow the wave to toss you about helplessly? No.

93

You observe the wave approaching, you bob along with it, and you allow it to pass.

Cravings are like that wave—or like that distraction—momentarily unsettling the steadiness of your effort. To try to stop it is a form of denial. The wave is coming, whether you like it or not. If you choose not to see it, it will slam you when you aren't looking. If you submit to it, it will carry you along uncontrollably until the next wave hits, and then the next.

A client of mine, Anita, a real estate agent in her mid-fifties (whom I had previously coached for nearly a year as she lost thirty pounds) was advised by her physician to reduce her salt intake to help control her elevated blood pressure. Both of Anita's parents had died of heart attacks in their early fifties, so Anita was sensitive to this issue and was committed to following her doctor's instructions. Though she had previously been a self-proclaimed "salt fiend," during our most recent round of coaching she chose to completely eliminate adding salt to her food, as well as all salty snacks and salty foods, such as cured meats and canned vegetables. And she rigorously cut back on foods that might have other forms of sodium "hidden" in them.

During our coaching calls, Anita often discussed her intense salt cravings, which of course started on the very day she chose to reduce salt. In the early going, she reported feeling frustrated because she could only hold off a craving for half an hour or so. Often she found herself bingeing on potato chips or salty pretzels before she even knew what hit her. "It's strange," she told me. "One second I'm fully aware of the craving and collecting my strength to overcome it, the next second I find myself sitting there chowing voraciously on chips."

Eventually she was able to resist the craving for more extended periods of time—several days. But the longer she resisted them, the more frequently they occurred, until she reached a point where she craved salt constantly. Ultimately she would give in, consuming considerably more salt than she normally would have. She had tried to resist the wave, and it swept her away.

Next, Anita decided she might crave salt because her body had a genuine physiological need for additional sodium. She was starting to anthropomorphize the craving, as if it were an animal that was living in her house, and she reasoned, "If I feed it a little, perhaps that will satisfy the hunger without doing the damage I've been doing by withholding from it and driving it crazy." So in essence, she had decided to submit to her craving.

Anita soon learned, however, that submitting to her craving in a controlled manner was not as easy as she had thought. Her craving's small feedings turned into huge feasts, and soon she found herself again almost-unknowingly devouring excessive amounts of salt.

Anita had exhausted what she saw as her only two options for coping with her cravings.

I knew from our history of coaching that Anita had made great progress in her practice of mindfulness. She was ready for the third option.

"The next time you get a salt craving, Anita," I suggested, "I'd like you to greet it without any intention to either resist it or give in to it. Simply observe it. Let it be a reminder for you to return to mindfulness of the present moment. Observe your breath, and observe the craving."

By the time we had our next coaching session two weeks later, Anita's salt cravings had disappeared.

"What happened?" I asked.

"I'm embarrassed to admit, it was easy," Anita said. "The night after our call, I had my usual strong salt craving. I simply sat down in a comfortable chair in my living room and tried to stay in the moment. I followed my breath, and I observed the craving. I greeted it like an old friend, just as you taught me to greet difficult emotions while practicing mindfulness. *'There you are, craving, my old friend. Nice to see you.'* After a few minutes, I set about doing my typical household evening tasks—paying bills, straightening up, and so forth. The craving passed."

But it wasn't over so soon, she reported. In the days following this initial success, Anita experienced more cravings. Often they were intense.

"I stayed in the moment with these cravings," she said. "I got curious about them. Where does the craving come from? Where does it go?"

After another few days, Anita's cravings started to seem less tangible to her. "I can't say it was all in my mind," she told me, "because those cravings were strong and very real. But, in a certain sense, I came to see that I was creating them."

But that wasn't the end of Anita's progression. "Several days ago, I was at a friend's house for dinner, and before our meal was ready, she set out a small bowl of salted nuts to snack on," Anita recalled. "Nuts have always been one of my favorite vehicles for salt, and as soon as I saw that bowl full of them, my craving surged. I remained mindful of it, staying conscious of my breathing and of this intense craving, which was leading to all sorts of physical sensations in my mouth and in my stomach. But the craving didn't let up. Finally, I chose to go ahead and eat a small handful of nuts. I stayed mindful of the taste of the salt and of my craving, and of the interplay between the two. In a way I can't describe, it seemed that the taste of salt suddenly had no relation to the craving. I had no problem stopping after that one handful of nuts, and I haven't had a craving since."

When Anita paid close enough attention, it turned out, she learned that her craving, when tended to, would blossom and then fade like a flower. Cravings have a dreamlike quality: They are real, but not as real as they may seem.

She rose above the common pitfall of listening to her craving, which often takes the form of thinking, *"I crave such-and-such, so I must genuinely need more of it."* Any recovering drug addict can testify that such a thought is delusional. (If you are hooked on an addictive substance—whether it be caffeine, nicotine, opium, or alcohol—there is no question that your craving can have a strong biochemical component and may require medical treatment. I believe that mindfulness can still be an essential skill for coping with these cravings; however, if addiction is an issue for you, consult your physician or an addiction counselor).

Anita kept me on as her coach for a long time as she continued to cultivate an advanced state of well-being. And she never had another salt craving. Her story perfectly exemplifies how mindfulness is the most effective tool for coping with cravings. The solution is neither in suppressing cravings nor in submitting to them. The solution is to be *aware* of them, without judging them, comparing them, or getting mired in them. Only then can you let your cravings go.

Once you are proficient at using mindfulness to cope with cravings related to your physical health, you will find that this skill is also useful in other areas of your life. After all, it is human nature to experience cravings, often on a scale much grander than simple salt cravings. You might crave wealth, stability, other people, change, security, power, perfection, knowledge, acceptance, vengeance, validation, fame, or even immortality. With mindfulness, you can attend to any of your cravings in a manner that is healthy for you and, in the process, allay your nagging feeling of deprivation.

❖

MIND YOUR CHANGE

The next time a craving arises in you, be mindful of it. Strive to bring your full attention to this craving at the earliest possible moment in its life—perhaps even before it is fully born, while it exists only as an impulse. Stay aware of your breath and, without getting lost in thought, bring your intuitive curiosity to your craving. What exactly is it? A feeling? A thought? A physical sensation? Where does it come from? Where does it go? If you keep a journal, write about your cravings for a period of at least three days.

EMBRACE CHOICELESSNESS

ACCEPTING that you are "at-choice" with your health—that it is a product of choices you have made—is an essential early step toward permanent change. Yet embracing *choicelessness* may prove to be your most rewarding strategy for reinforcing new behaviors.

This is not a contradiction, as my client Nathan, a forty-three-year-old businessman from Dallas, learned while transforming from a wellness wannabe into a highly fit and satisfied health seeker. Nathan's initial goal was to exercise at his health club after work four days a week. But time and time again, as he drove away from his office—his energy draining as he sat in stop-and-go traffic, half-listening to talk radio—he found himself turning away from the club and choosing to drive home. He surrendered to the pull of a comforting dinner, chit-chat with the family, and a couple of hours "vegging out" in front of the television.

Nathan felt conflicted. He genuinely wanted to get into better shape, and he didn't mind exercising, but day after day he made that turn—both literally and figuratively—away from exercise and toward the comfort of home.

I offered Nathan three suggestions:

- At the beginning of each week, decide which four days you will work out on, and note them as appointments in your daily calendar.

- Change into your workout clothes before leaving work.

- E-mail me each day when you get home from the club to let me know how your workout went.

Each of these suggestions, which I have used to great effect with hordes of aspiring exercisers, was designed to reduce Nathan's inclination to make an impulsive choice to skip his workout. By scheduling exercise into his week, and adding an element of accountability by reporting in to me, Nathan was less likely to view *not* exercising as an option.

When health seekers plan to work out a certain number of days per week and then wait until each day to decide whether that particular one will be a workout day, the slightest temptation to choose an easier, more comfortable course leads them to think, *"No, I'll exercise tomorrow, or some other day, instead."* At that point, they are making a choice. By scheduling their workouts in advance, they eliminate the opportunity to choose. Nathan, for example, incorporated as an ordinary part of his life an exercise schedule that included Mondays, Tuesdays, Thursdays, and Fridays. Plain and simple. There was no sitting in his car, thinking, *"Should I work out, or shouldn't I?"*

Nathan solidified his choicelessness by changing into his workout apparel prior to leaving the office. It was his way of saying to himself that the choice was already made, before he lost his momentum while sitting in traffic.

Ultimately, Nathan achieved a high level of fitness that he maintains to this day.

Choicelessness is a key ingredient for weight-loss success, as well, and it is one of the reasons health seekers can lose weight on almost any diet. Health seekers living in a relatively prosperous society are overwhelmed these days by food choices. Enter a supermarket and you are bombarded by displays of tempting foods; the media constantly tempt you with articles and advertisements for snacks you absolutely must try; coworkers offer bowls of candy at work, visitors bring you food as gifts, restaurants offer larger and larger selections of culinary delights served in colossal portions. These are all choices that are put before you, and any health seeker who experiences the slightest moment of weakness no doubt will have a tempting but less-than-healthful food choice available when that moment arrives.

But when you commit to a diet, you say, *"I am going to limit my choices."* And, frankly, it can make your life a lot easier. You come to see that the abundance of food that has always surrounded you actually leads to stress and confusion. The choices have been overwhelming. When you diet, you limit them and gain control.

When coaching health seekers who wish to lose weight, I use choice-limiting strategies similar to those that worked so well for Nathan as he was shaping up. I encourage weekly meal planning—including scheduling specific meals, in writing, on their calendars (many dieters already are doing this). And since health seekers on diets often fret about food-centered social events, such as parties or receptions, I advise them to find out in advance what will be served, or what the menu options will be. Then they can decide beforehand what they will eat. Indeed, choicelessness often entails making your choices in advance—circumventing the opportunity to be driven by impulsiveness—rather than not making any choice at all. This rigorous adherence to planning may not sound like your idea of a good time, but dieters who are genuinely committed to weight loss report that it sharply reduces the stress in their lives. Even if they choose to indulge a little, they proceed knowing that they have purposefully built a treat into their plan, rather than simply surrendering to impulse.

You create ease in your life when you take a straightforward path with as few forks in the road as possible. But even paths that appear straightforward may sometimes have a Möbius-strip quality—perhaps not diverging, but instead turning inside out. Choosing choicelessness is one such path. It seems contradictory, but it's not.

You are still "at-choice." You simply choose to establish a boundary around your options—one of the most empowering actions you can take. When you do so, you will experience a multifold increase in your health confidence, your well-being, and, as a result, your overall sense of inner strength.

Mind Your Change

If you have created a living environment that supports your health change (see the "Change Your World" chapter), you may already have embraced choicelessness. Either way, revisit your environment, paying special attention to choicelessness. If you wish to improve your eating habits, remove unhealthful food options from your cupboards. If you're embarking on an exercise program, schedule your workouts in your calendar—and also schedule your most enticing diversions, such as television, leisure reading, work, and home improvement projects, so you won't impulsively choose them over exercise. If you're quitting cigarettes, remove from your environment not only all tobacco products, but anything that triggers you to smoke, such as coffee or alcoholic beverages.

Use your imagination. You have unlimited choices in your life. Consequently, you have unlimited opportunities to embrace choicelessness.

Six Focal Points
to Keep You On Track

Oₙ‌E of the main reasons people hire coaches is to help them stay focused. A good coach will keep you on track using a number of techniques, not the least of which is simple goal setting and accountability. But one of my favorites is what I like to call "pinpoint questions."

Frequently, health seekers have so many goals, so many obstacles, so many resources, or so many plans that they don't know where to start. Or, to put it more accurately, they can think of too many places to start: They start x, then they start y, then they start z. Before they know it, they've long forgotten x. Ultimately, they can't make progress with anything because as soon as they start one thing, they drop it like a hot potato and start something else—a new goal or a different strategy. In the end, they criticize themselves for procrastinating when in fact their problem is not that they are delaying, but that they are over-responding.

Ask yourself the following pinpoint questions about your health change:

1. What is the one action you can take today that will move you closer to your goal?

2. Who is the one person in your life who can support you the most?

3. What is your one most intimidating obstacle?

4. What is your one greatest strength, and how will you use it to achieve your goal?

5. What is the one most significant accomplishment of your life, and what was the lesson you learned from that accomplishment that will help you with your current endeavor?

6. What is the number-one reason you want to attain this goal?

Of course, this list could go on and on. But I limit it to six because if it gets too long, these focal points can, rather than keeping you on track, just be another set of distractions that can derail you.

MIND YOUR CHANGE
Bring your health change into perfect focus by answering, in one word (okay, I'll cut you some slack: fewer than five words), question number one from the preceding list: What is the one action you can take today?
    Take it.

Multiple Changes

A couple of years ago I planted two trees. In my backyard, I planted a lovely gingko—its simple, fan-shaped leaves evoking the gentle grace found in many Japanese gardens. In the front, I planted an emerald maple, the tallest and most classical element in my garden.

I was reminded of these trees recently when a client asked me whether it was better to change one health habit at a time or to change several simultaneously.

It's a wonderful question, one that I think many of us ponder at some time. Smokers, it's worth noting, are usually advised not to diet while quitting tobacco. In fact, cessation counselors advise smokers to be prepared to gain ten pounds or so. "Focus on quitting smoking," they say. "In the long run, smoking is much more deleterious to your health than that extra ten pounds." (Noble advice, but small consolation in a fat-phobic society in which appearance is valued as much, if not more, than long-term health. Many smokers, especially young women, identify weight maintenance as one of the main reasons they smoke in the first place!)

On the other hand, if someone has an array of unhealthy habits and is diagnosed with, say, diabetes or heart disease, generally they'll be advised to stop smoking, start exercising, lose weight, adopt a healthy diet—everything, now.

But if you have the choice, do you start with one habit or target a few? Do you conduct a clean sweep, simultaneously addressing each and every aspect of your life that you feel is not up to par? And what if your behaviors are intertwined, as diet and exercise are for health seekers who wish to lose weight?

These are the questions I contemplated one recent autumn as I enjoyed observing my trees. The gingko leaves had turned a bright yellow, and from a distance the young tree's form resembled that of a lit candle. One mid-October night, the temperature sank below freezing for the first time that year, and the following morning all the leaves fell from the tree—every last one. Only their outlines remained on the frosty ground below after the leaves were swept away by the wind.

The emerald maple led a different kind of life. Through the course of the season, its foliage gradually turned from green to fiery red, and finally brown. Then it began to let go of its tenacious leaves one by one, thinning gradually throughout October, until it was completely bare around the week before Thanksgiving.

One type of tree turned its leaves and shed them all at once; the other took its time and let them go one by one.

I have searched the scientific literature high and low to find out what the research says about which is more effective—changing multiple health behaviors in synchronicity or addressing them individually across time—only to learn that there are no surefire answers yet.

But in my experience as a coach, I have found that health seekers make changes just as those trees do. Some do best when their changes take place singularly. For others, transitions flow most naturally when they all are undertaken concurrently. Either way, the important thing is to be firmly rooted, well supported, and adequately nourished, and to grow stronger, rather than whither, while yielding to harsh but ever-changing conditions.

MIND YOUR CHANGE

For health seekers who require more definitive guidance, it may be helpful to think of health change as a zero-sum game. Smokers are advised not to diet while engaged in quitting, it's true; on the other hand, they are urged to exercise. One reason for this is that it's often beneficial to replace behaviors you are giving up with new, healthier behaviors.

If you think of each newly adopted behavior as +1, and each dropped behavior as -1, you can see that quitting tobacco (-1) and starting exercise (+1) cancel each other out and equal zero. So there's an intrinsic balance that many health seekers find easier to maintain.

Another example is diet (-1) and exercise (+1): a zero sum and therefore, for many, a natural complement. Compare that to initiating an exercise program (+1) and initiating a meditation program (+1). That yields a sum of +2—piling it on rather than striking a balance. Similarly, giving up caffeine (-1) and cutting back on sweets (-1) equals -2—likely overextending and, again, compounding the challenges.

This is an individual matter, but you will undoubtedly gain insight from exploring this zero-sum perspective. Consider: What is the sum of *your* health changes?

Part III
Chill Out

JUST DO IT...SOME OTHER TIME

ALEXIA is a single mom. Working and parenting keep her on the go. All her time is devoted to things like cooking meals, shuttling the kids to after-school programs, and participating in the PTA, not to mention commuting, managing the household, and trying to carve out at least a few minutes for herself.

Margaret is a different story. Her kids are grown and out of the house, and her husband shares in the household chores. But at work, she's committed for the next six weeks to a team that's putting together a proposal for an important client. The whole team works late every night, and Margaret is exhausted by the time she gets home, with just enough energy for a few minutes of relaxing one-on-one time with her spouse.

Both Margaret and Alexia feel like they're letting their wellness get away from them. They want to eat better, exercise more, and have less stress.

I often speak to health seekers about the need to prioritize and give up something in their lives in order to create space for change. How can Alexia and Margaret do that?

I'm sure my answer is quite different from anything the "media experts" will tell you. Even most coaches would assert that these two women are "running on adrenaline" and need to make immediate changes. This *may* be true. For example, if Alexia can call upon friends or family to help out with the kids, she'll gain time for herself. But is it in her best interest to fill this newly created gap with, say, scheduled exercise? That wouldn't be *creating* space; it would be *trading* space—a pitfall to be wary of.

The point is, Alexia *has* prioritized: Her priority just happens to be her kids. This state of affairs will last a long time, but not forever. Margaret may have bitten off more at work than she can chew—and may be neglecting to stake her claim to wellness because of it—but only for a finite period of time. This simply may not be the right time for Alexia or Margaret to introduce health changes into their hectic lives.

We need to recognize that there are cycles in our lives, and certain cycles are more suited to health change than others. For now, Alexia and Margaret can focus on optimizing the circumstances they have and devising a long-term plan so they can see the light at the end of the tunnel. They may even choose to set goals for when they *will* introduce health changes into their lives, regardless of whether those changes are a few weeks or a few years away.

I'm the first person to encourage health seekers to slow down and to simplify. But I also recognize that you may find yourself at a stage of life in which you cannot slow down. This must be respected. Aren't you better off focusing on what needs to be done now, and then advancing to what's next in life, rather than trying to do it all today—work, fitness, family, diet, art, spiritual practice, volunteerism—only to become overwhelmed and disheartened?

Sometimes health seekers are best served by embracing the cycles of their lives and getting in sync with them. This is an important method to facilitate the flow of energy in life and to reduce resistance to that flow. Of course this doesn't apply to changes that have clear and immediate medical implications: If your doctor tells you to reduce your blood pressure now, then do it now.

I'm not necessarily giving you the nod to say to yourself, *"He's right, this just isn't the right time for me to exercise. I'm too busy."* The fact is, most people do need to slow down and take better care of themselves. But not everyone is in a position to do so at any given time.

MIND YOUR CHANGE

In your journal, draw or paint a picture that depicts the path your life has taken, from birth to the present, and beyond (if you wish). Use colors and textures if you can, but don't delay because you don't have the right materials. Make do with whatever you have lying around: paints, crayons, pencils, markers. Have fun with this and let yourself go. Don't censor or concern yourself with artistic quality. Make it free-flowing. You can use this type of activity to see the full picture of your life—what has happened, what will happen, the types of changes that could only take place concurrently, and the types that required singular focus. There are patterns and characteristics in your life. Look for them. You will come to see that your path is not as linear as it may seem, and that with creative planning, you can accomplish what you wish to, without the pressure to do it all right now.

HIT THAT SNOOZE BUTTON

A LOT of health seekers decide that early morning is the time for action. They vow to wake up an hour earlier to work out, or to meditate, or to prepare a healthy lunch to take to work. Is this a good strategy? Generally, you have better options.

There are at least two big problems with the crack-of-dawn strategy:

1. If you were really that much of a morning person, you'd already be up at that time. You *need* that sleep. It is as important a part of your health as whatever it is you're sacrificing it for—probably more important. Studies have shown that getting an average of seven hours of sleep per night or less is correlated with increased risk of heart disease.

2. Over and over again I've seen that when health seekers start waking up earlier, especially to do something they find laborious, they gradually revert to their old routine— sleeping until their usual time and foregoing their newly adopted healthy lifestyle. Inevitably, they chalk this up as a failure. "I started going for walks in the morning," they may say, "but I couldn't stick with it," or, "I was going great preparing healthy lunches for work, then I stopped." But they may not know what really set them back. They assume it was the health practice. But I estimate that, 95 percent of the time, it's the sleep deprivation.

You may hear that people who work out in the early morning are the ones most likely to stick with it for the long term. But a lot of these early risers were already up at that hour, anyway, and decided to fill the time with exercise—they didn't just suddenly "discover" they only needed six hours of sleep a night, when all their lives it felt like they needed seven or eight.

So if you really are an early bird, sitting around at five a.m. twiddling your thumbs, by all means consider it a fine time to do your health-related activities. But if you prefer to slumber in your warm and cozy bed at that hour, then go ahead and hit that snooze button.

What are your options? Remember the chapter "How to Make Health Fit"? When you take on something big in your life, such as a health change, you have to free up time and energy in order to make it possible. You can do that by letting go of projects and other goals. Sleep deprivation does not create space; it creates a deficit.

MIND YOUR CHANGE

This week, you won't have to worry about the snooze on your alarm clock because you're not going to set your alarm.

That's right: For the next seven days, wake up without any assistance from external beeps, bells, or buzzes. It's a fail-safe way to make sure you're getting the z's you need.

And if you're worried you won't wake up early enough to be on time for your first commitment of the day, then there is *one* thing you can plan on doing earlier—going to bed.

Pssst! Is Your Wellness Classified?

Often health seekers keep their health-change efforts a big secret. They don't tell their friends, their coworkers, or their spouse about the improvement they're trying to make.

Generally, you stamp your health change as CLASSIFIED for at least one of three reasons:

1. You're looking for dramatic effect, anticipating the day when people start commenting on how much you've changed, how much better you look, or how a bright light follows you wherever you go. If you're trying to lose weight, you may fantasize about people exclaiming, "Wow! You look terrific! What's your secret?" or a simple, "Honey, have you lost weight?" And, indeed, if you do lose weight, your friends and family may very well shower you with praise.

   Behind this desire for dramatic effect often lies a deeper, underlying need for approval. Nothing unusual about that. In fact, I find that much of what drives most health seekers is a need for approval. This is why coaches spend a lot of time working with clients around "needs"—not just the need for approval, but other needs, such as control, power, security, love, and meaning. Usually, we coaches don't encourage clients to eliminate their needs; we encourage them to set up systems to get those needs met.

   Health seekers get better results when their health changes are motivated by growth and self-care, rather than when they are part of an everlasting effort to satisfy a long-unfulfilled need.

2. Another rationale for health-change stealth—perhaps the prevalent rationale—is that if you don't tell anyone you're trying to make a change, then you don't have to tell anyone if you fail.

3. A final reason you may conduct your change as a clandestine operation is that it requires a financial commitment, perhaps a health club membership, weight-loss program dues, or coaching fees, and you do not want others (this most commonly is a secret kept from spouses) to know about the expense. In my opinion, this is a dynamic that usually has far-reaching and deep-seated implications for a relationship, way beyond the scope of coaching. When clients confide to me that they don't want their spouse to know how much they're investing in their health, I almost always refer them to couples counseling.

I urge health seekers to be open about health changes. The advantage of dropping the veil of secrecy is that it allows you to put into play two must-have strategies:

1. *Asking for help.* The support of others is a key component to successful change. And usually you'll have to ask for this support, rather than just passively waiting for it to appear. Either way, you'll never get the support you need if you don't tell anyone what you're up to.

2. *Staking your claim to better health.* You have a right to establish boundaries that prohibit others from undermining your efforts. But you have a responsibility to make those

boundaries known. How do you do this if you're conducting a clandestine operation?

My client Cheryl, a thirty-something homemaker, told me she had once set a date for herself to give up junk food as part of her commitment to losing weight. She didn't mention anything to her husband, Ian. About a week after her "quit date," Ian came home from work with a small bag and, sporting an eager grin, announced to Cheryl that he had brought home for dessert a pint of specialty ice cream and all the fixings for sundaes! Whipped cream, chocolate syrup, maraschino cherries—the whole kit and kaboodle. Cheryl felt put on the spot. She knew Ian anticipated a grateful response, and it felt like the wrong time to tell him she had given up such indulgent culinary atrocities seven days before. So after dinner that night, beset with feelings of guilt and overall confusion, she and Ian shared the mother of all sundaes.

Thus ended that round of Cheryl's junk food renunciation. What's more, for several weeks she blamed Ian for the whole imbroglio. She loved him, but if he hadn't undermined her that night she never would have touched ice cream again in her life and no doubt would have been well on her way to prodigious weight loss and celestial perfection.

Fortunately, Cheryl had a high level of self-awareness, and over time she came to realize that Ian was innocent. He didn't know she had elected to forego junk food, and in fact his gesture that night had been filled with caring and love. When Cheryl finally discussed her wellness ambitions with Ian, he readily directed his loving nature to providing Cheryl with unconditional support.

Needs, fears, support, boundaries: This is the stuff of *real* health transformation. And that's why mere willpower or simplistic goal-and-reward strategies don't make the grade, and why more whole person–oriented approaches, such as those you're reading about in this handbook, bear real results.

Mind Your Change

Are you working on a personal health change in secret? Maybe you're just mentioning it to a few select people? Think of someone close to you whom you've decided not to tell. What do you gain from this secretiveness? Would it be helpful to get this person's support, or to set a boundary? Come out of the wellness closet today.

Skip the Planning
and the Preparation

Sometimes health seekers should skip their planning and their preparations and just take the plunge.

For example, last spring my client Nan told me she had always wanted to run a 10K (a 6.2-mile foot race). And since she had hardly run at all since she had given birth to her son three years before, she believed that entering a race would motivate her to stick to a consistent training schedule. Nan had a particular race in mind, but before actually registering she wanted to run regularly for a month to prove to herself that she was up to the task. In other words, Nan was afraid she might enter the race, then never actually get around to training fully, and ultimately fail.

"What I want for you," I told Nan, "is to register for the race today."

You see, Nan was caught in a Catch-22: She wanted to enter the race so she would have a goal that motivated her, but she needed to feel more motivated before she could bring herself to commit to the race. We can languish in such Catch-22s indefinitely. So I helped her convert her dilemma into what I call a "Coach-22."

Nan took the plunge and entered the race. I coached her quite a bit around managing her time to allow for training, soliciting help from her husband to share more of the household and child-care tasks, and creating space in her life so she had the energy to train and stay motivated. We did some peak performance coaching, as well, in which Nan visualized herself running the course. When race day came around and she proudly crossed that finish line—greeted by her cheering husband and little boy—her mind was clear and her body well tuned.

Nan's behavioral change had ramifications far beyond her physical health. In a coaching session that took place well after she had run the race, I asked Nan to make a list of ten other goals in her life that she was forestalling until a time when all conditions were perfect. Prior to our next session, she e-mailed me a list of twenty-five such goals! She is now well on her way to achieving most of them.

There are two lessons health seekers can learn from Nan's experience:

1. Skip the planning and the preparation. I won't say, "Just do it." But I will say, "Start today."

2. When you identify hindrances that hold you back from making a change, take a look and acknowledge the other areas of your life where they may be limiting you.

MIND YOUR CHANGE
Consider a health goal—such as losing weight, getting fit, or reducing stress—and identify the one thing that most stands in your way. Now, list ten other goals in your life that are on hold due to the same impediment. At this point, I'm not asking you to commit to working on these goals—that will only inhibit you from listing them all. Just list them.

Believe This

It's often said that our beliefs can shape our health. But from a coaching perspective, the more important point is that our beliefs shape the *actions* we take related to our health. Certain beliefs lead to healthy actions; others lead to unhealthy actions. Certain beliefs are correct; others may not be.

If you want to modify your lifestyle, including your health habits and other behaviors, then you may have to shift your beliefs.

In previous chapters, I touched on specific types of beliefs that shape health. For example, the more health confidence you have—your confidence in your own ability to change a health behavior—the more likely you are to succeed with your health change. This means that you hold the belief *"I will do it"* versus the belief *"I can't do it,"* or the even more damning *"It can't be done."*

"I can't do it" is a perfect example of a limiting belief. But so is *"It can't be done."* Limiting beliefs can be about the way things are; they may not necessarily be about the belief owner, specifically. Transforming limiting beliefs is often an important part of the coaching process.

Here are examples of common limiting beliefs. Reflect on whether any of these are included in your own belief system:

- I deserve to be unhealthy.

- There aren't enough hours in the day.

- If I want to make a change, I need to have the will. It starts here.

- If I want to make a change, I need the help of a professional, or a pill. It starts there.

- A good change strategy will lead to quick results.

- A good change strategy requires sacrifice.

- People don't change.

- You can't teach an old dog new tricks.

- There are unknown powers at work keeping me this way.

- I'm this way because of my parents.

- Whatever can go wrong will go wrong.

- With my luck... (Why doesn't anyone ever say, "With my luck, something really great is bound to happen!")

The connection between beliefs and health behaviors has been well established by health and psychology researchers. Indeed, one of the few theories developed specifically to understand health behavior, as opposed to more general theories of behavior that have been recast to apply to health, is the Health Belief Model, which has been studied extensively and has been widely accepted over the past fifty years.

The Health Belief Model postulates that health seekers will take action to prevent illness, to participate in a screening, or to manage a disease if they believe that:

- They are at risk of getting sick or sicker.

- Not taking action will have a severe impact on their health and their life.

- The courses of action available to them will effectively reduce the threat of illness.

- The barriers to change, such as inconvenience, expense, or discomfort, are outweighed by the benefits.

The Health Belief Model was originally developed by the brilliant social psychologist Godfrey Hochbaum, who was called upon by the U.S. Public Health Service to figure out why free, government-sponsored mobile tuberculosis screenings attracted few participants. This was during an era when tuberculosis was a much bigger problem than it is today.

Of course the model doesn't explain all health seekers' motivations under all circumstances. It's unclear whether the model applies when your ultimate goal is not health related but is a measure of something else. For example, if you're trying to lose weight in order to improve your appearance, the issue of susceptibility to illness doesn't seem directly relevant. As you consider your personal circumstances, however, you undoubtedly will find applications for the Health Belief Model.

Let's say you're going to start a walking program to lose weight. You may wish to ask yourself whether you truly believe you can achieve significant long-term weight loss by walking. I know you can, but do *you* believe it? If you don't, then you may hold the limiting belief "Walking won't work for weight loss."

Here are three tips for avoiding and shifting limiting beliefs:

1. *Your language is influenced by your beliefs, but your beliefs are also manifestations of your language.* If you have identified a belief that you would like to shift, use affirmations. For example, if you are stuck in that oldie but goody "My parents made me this way," use an affirmation like "I have the power to change!" (Notice the positive tone of the affirmation, as opposed to, say, "This problem is my own fault.") You can start by simply writing this message on a sticky-note and posting it on the mirror you use in the morning as you get ready for the day. But ultimately you should start saying the message aloud, at least once daily. Most health seekers feel silly when they first start saying affirmations aloud—although, unfortunately, they're all too comfortable saying negative things to themselves—but you get used to it. And simply getting more comfortable with saying good things that expand your beliefs is a step in the right direction.

2. *Be wary of dogma.* Dogma generally represents a systemized structure of limiting beliefs. If you are attached to any particular dogma that you do not want to let go of, at least investigate it. Consider the tenets of your dogma—whether it's related to your work, your spiritual belief, or anything else in your life—and be aware of the possibilities that are being ruled out.

3. *Be open, and educate yourself about beliefs that are different from yours.* I'll give you an example from my own life: I've always believed that high-protein, low-carbohydrate diets are misguided, and I've said so in my newsletters and presentations. My disdain for these diets was fueled by much of the

scientific literature I read. More recently, however, as I have continued to educate myself, my respect for the pro-protein movement has increased dramatically. I'm not quite ready to do infomercials for them. But I do believe that evidence has been shifting in favor of high-protein diets. And certainly I have shifted my own eating practices as a result.

This is a great time to flex your letting-go muscle. Leave your limiting beliefs behind you. You may just find yourself entering a new world—one of unlimited possibilities.

MIND YOUR CHANGE

Every "should" is built on a belief. Many coaches advise their clients never to utter the word "should." I'm not that draconian. But I do recommend that you exercise mindfulness in your use of the word. Today, note how many times you use the word *should*. Each time you find yourself using it, take a moment to identify the underlying belief. Then determine whether this belief helps you or hinders you.

You're Not a Lazybones

When I coach health seekers, I don't tell them they're wrong, or make them feel wrong about anything, because generally I think people are not wrong about themselves. One of my golden rules of coaching is that clients are the foremost experts on themselves.

But there's one exception: When clients tell me they are procrastinators, or just plain lazy, I do tell them they're wrong. Or I'm more likely to say, in my most coachy tone, "You may perceive yourself as a procrastinator, but I believe you're not."

You see, when you call yourself a procrastinator or a lazybones, not only are you invoking one of the world's foremost self-limiting beliefs, but you also are making a declaration that isn't true.

You are not a procrastinator! You are not lazy! Sure, at times you may have delayed (perhaps indefinitely) taking an action. But there are many reasons why this happens, and most of them are not a reflection of who you are.

Let's say you intend to get a gym membership but you keep putting it off. Does this warrant labeling yourself as a procrastinator, a self-classification that will undermine you in every aspect of your life? No.

- Perhaps you're not getting the gym membership because you have no confidence that you'll follow through with it.

- Perhaps, when you get right down to the nitty-gritty, working out at a gym just doesn't seem like "you."

- Maybe you're encountering fear: of failure, of looking goofy, or of something else.

- Or maybe your gym-membership goal is just as stale and rank as an old sweat sock.

Procrastination and laziness? These are symptoms.

Often, I find, clients think of themselves as procrastinators or as lazy because someone else has identified them as such, often a long, long time ago. It may have been a teacher. A parent. A spouse.

But remember, you came into this world with boundless energy and unlimited potential. That potential still lives within you.

So please, don't tell me that you're a procrastinator or you're lazy. It will be my duty to inform you that you're wrong.

Mind Your Change

Today, choose two actions you have been putting off for a long time. Do one of them. See if there's another one you can resolve *not* to do. And let it go.

THE BRIGHTER SIDE OF NEGATIVE THINKING

In a previous chapter, "The Perils of Positive Thinking," I described the foibles of positive thinkers and offered five suggestions for cultivating genuine positivism to keep you moving forward in your life. Of course at the opposite end of the spectrum from positive thinkers are those people who tend to view the world with a negative bias. You probably know people whom you consider to be negative. They are always complaining: wishing they had a better job, seeing the worst in themselves and in others, griping incessantly about the government.

Occasionally, these negative types show up for health coaching, most commonly in corporate programs where they perceive that they are pressured to enroll or where they've been given some incentive to participate. Clients like this represent a unique challenge for a coach.

I myself have developed a soft spot for negative thinkers. Western society (more so than people in other parts of the world) is so strongly biased in favor of high-energy, positive people that negative types come to feel ostracized. In reality, they often are sensitive people who are highly attuned to what's going on around them. Recent research has even shown that, when recalling past experiences, negative thinkers are actually less biased than positive thinkers; that is, they tend to be more accurate in their recollections, rather than distorting the facts to paint a prettier picture.

And negative thinkers *are* ostracized. As a result, they make their best effort to bottle up their frustrations and their discontent; however, in many cases, it comes out despite their most valiant efforts because expressing themselves negatively is the only way they know. This bottling up allows their negativity to fester, and so they find themselves entangled in a cycle that offers them limited means of escape.

I coached a client, Kevin, who worked as a systems engineer for a large financial company that had hired me. On our first coaching call, his tone of voice smacked of indifference and I deduced that he was ambivalent about being coached and may have resented the role I had been asked to play. This didn't exactly seem like a formula for success. Kevin did, however, want to lose weight. And he proclaimed to me that he would be the most challenging client I had ever had.

It turns out that part of the reason Kevin's health confidence was so low was that he had already spent a small fortune on weight-loss schemes, yet he continued to put on pounds. He had tried chromium picolinate, fasting shakes, celebrity diet books, and every other quick fix you can name. When I broached the subject of exercise, he wanted no part of it. He hated exercise and in fact couldn't see himself taking up healthy eating either. He loved red meat, pizza, cheese, ice cream, and all that good stuff.

Yowza. Well, over a period of several weeks I whipped out every trick I had in my coaching hat. And repeatedly he came back to our coaching sessions telling me why whatever he had agreed to do the previous week turned out not to work or really wasn't feasible.

Finally, I offered him a focusing pinpoint question: "Kevin," I asked, "what is the one major reason that you can identify to justify *not* making lifestyle changes, such as exercise, that will help you attain this goal?"

Kevin thought for a long time. Finally, he said, "Well, I can't narrow it down to one reason. I have so many. I could write ten pages full of reasons."

"Go ahead and do that, then," I quickly replied.

"What?"

"Do that as this week's fieldwork. Write ten pages in your journal on why you can't or shouldn't exercise. If you haven't kept a journal as we discussed in the early going, don't worry about it. Any notebook or paper will do." I was following a hunch.

"Well," Kevin argued, "I can come up with ten pages about why I shouldn't do *that!*"

"I'm sure you can, Kevin. But you came to coaching for a reason. I know no one is forcing you to do it. You've told me you'd like to make a change. Somewhere along the line, you have to take *some* action. So this is the action I am asking you to take right now. And though you may not be able to appreciate its value, I request that you do this even if that means making a leap of faith."

At our next session, Kevin reported that he had done his ten pages.

"Read them to me," I said.

Kevin sighed. I could tell he was getting exasperated. But underneath it all he was a kind, cooperative fellow, and so he started reading. He read to me about how much he hated exercise, how boring it was, how much it hurt the next day, how people who exercised were obsessed with their bodies, how there wasn't enough time, how there were no gyms near him and no space in his house for equipment, how he felt stupid walking for exercise in his neighborhood, and how sometimes there was

131

bad weather, and exercise just made him hungry. Around page six, he stopped and said to me, "Some of this sounds pretty ridiculous, doesn't it?"

"Not ridiculous," I said.

"Well, I don't want to read any more," he said.

"Okay," I replied. "Thank you for doing the work and for reading to me what you did."

"I suppose now I'm supposed to magically start exercising or something?" he said.

"Do you want to?" I asked.

There was a long pause. Remember, we were on the phone, and if you haven't experienced a quiet pause of thirty seconds or more on the phone, you'd be amazed at just how long it feels. We stayed there, quietly connected via fiber-optic cable. I could hear, outside my office, the sound of light traffic and, inside, the whirring fan in my computer printer and ever-so-faint hum of my monitor.

Kevin, I knew, had his own faint sounds that, right at that moment, probably seemed louder and clearer than ever.

Finally, he said, "I guess I should try."

That week Kevin started walking three days a week for twenty minutes. Eventually, he walked nearly every day for longer periods of time.

In the months I coached Kevin, he had more than his share of fits and starts. But that was an improvement over where he began. He had come to see his resistance to exercise for exactly what it was: resistance. And his periods of inactivity grew shorter and less frequent.

What exactly happened to Kevin, our negative thinker, in writing and reading those ten pages? Was the simple act of confronting his resistance enough to make it dissolve? No, it was more than that. Kevin needed to air out his resistance—to exorcise it, so to speak. He was a perfect example of someone who, though he often came off to others as negative, still had much of his negativity bottled up inside him and was unable to tune in to his positive wavelength as long as it was overshadowed by this pent-up negativity.

Be receptive to expressions of negativity as well as positivism. And be careful of what you label as negative thought, in yourself or in others. Do you remember the children's fairy tale *The Emperor's New Clothes?* A rich and powerful emperor is tricked into thinking he has been given a fine set of new clothes, though he is unable to see it. All the villagers support his delusion, acting as if he is wearing clothes and complimenting him on them. But one little boy cries out, "Why, the Emperor isn't wearing any clothes at all!" All the villagers then realize their folly and laugh at the Emperor, who realizes his folly, as well. These days, that little boy would be branded for not having a positive attitude—for being a negative thinker. We see this in the workplace time and time again. Employees support organizational strategies they know are misguided, for fear of being branded—not just by their boss but by their peers—as naysayers. How many organizations have gone belly up, and how many employees have suffered, because no one had the courage to risk appearing negative?

I love negative thinkers. They stand up and speak out. In fact, we owe much to people who are blessed with the combination of being highly critical and having superior problem-solving skills. They're the ones who can look around, see what's wrong, and make an improvement, whether it's a better way to do business, a new medical procedure, or simply a better mousetrap. If you believe that negative thinkers are all underachievers, contemplate whether that's an accurate assessment...or more a reflection of your own biases.

But don't get me wrong: People with chronically negative thinking patterns may really be suffering in their lives and may need professional help. It is likely that they have been traumatized in their life and still haven't healed. And certainly I don't recommend that people think *more* negatively.

But negative thinkers should be embraced—and if you are prone to thinking negatively, I urge you to embrace yourself, too. Negativity is part of the balance in our world. Negative thinkers are not negative people. They are doing much of our world's most difficult introspection. Many coaches advise their clients to avoid negative people, saying that such people will bring them down. Seems a bit misanthropic to me. Let's all embrace each other—health seekers who are negative, positive, neutral, and even those who run hot and cold. Let us all bring each other up. We need each other to reach our fullest potential. You need me, and I need you.

MIND YOUR CHANGE
Are you in the process of making a health change? Considering it? Fill ten pages of your journal with all the reasons not to. Start writing whatever you can come up with—what you may fear about your health change, what's stupid about it,

why it won't work—without allowing your intellect to self-censor it for any reason. Write, write, write. Then, and only then, write all the reasons why your health change is a positive step.

Identifying the positive certainly will support your success. But sometimes you first need to work through the negative.

Untie Your Knots; Or, Willpower Won't Power

On a warm day early one spring, I had a burst of energy and decided to water my garden for the first time that year. My garden hose had spent the winter hibernating twisted and tangled in some neighboring brush, so I reached into the brush, grabbed the end of the hose, and pulled it over to the spigot on the side of my house.

Turning the faucet, I heard a brief rush of water, but only for a moment before I felt the hose swelling as the pressure built inside it. *"That shouldn't happen,"* I thought. Since there was no nozzle at the other end of the hose, the water should have flowed freely. I turned the faucet on the spigot further, but the hose just grew fatter. Finally, I cranked that faucet all the way. Nothing.

Mystified, I followed the hose back to its other end, which still lay in the brush. Pushing the brush aside, I saw that there was a big knot near the end of the hose that was causing it to kink. The water could not pass. I untied the knot, and the water rushed through (spraying all over my face and clothes, naturally).

That evening, I reflected on how this entire garden hose entanglement was the perfect allegory for how to deal with resistance when making health changes:

- The water flowing—or not flowing—through the hose is like your health change.

- The knot is the obstacle that keeps your health change from flowing (often such obstacles reside in your personal "blind spot").

- The faucet represents your willpower. No matter how hard you try to blast through that knot, force alone isn't going to make it happen.

And you can't go around the knot either. You must untie it.

I'll even take the allegory one step further and suggest to you that clearing the brush is like practicing mindfulness—full attention to the present moment. Mindfulness clears the brush—that is, the overgrowth in your fertile mind—allowing what's really there to reveal itself to you, knots and all.

What, specifically in *your* life, does the knot represent? What obstacle impedes the flow of your health change? It may be anything, ranging from simple lack of confidence to childhood trauma.

You have many strategies available to untie your knots—therapy, reiki, spiritual practice, and, of course, coaching, to name a few. Your choice will depend on your own preferences and the nature of the obstacle.

But recognize this: Willpower, while it may play a role, is rarely an effective strategy in and of itself. More and more power is often met by more and more resistance. So be careful: If all you do is try to "will" your way through resistance, you may just blow a gasket.

Mind Your Change
Sometimes other people can see the resistance that hides in your blind spot. Ask someone close to you: "I'm trying to make such-and-such a change. Do you have any ideas about

why it's such a struggle for me?" Not comfortable doing this? Ask yourself why. Recognize that the knots that create resistance in one part of your life are the same knots that create resistance in other parts.

MOMENTS OF TRUTH

HEALTH seekers sometimes get hung up for years on a particular goal without making any headway. In cases like this it may take a flash of unbridled honesty—a moment of truth—to get them "unstuck."

Moments of truth occasionally spring up on their own, but not too often—the health seeker is too entrenched. More frequently these moments are evoked when the health seeker is forced to confront something dramatic in his or her life: loss of a loved one, a sudden reminder of a behavior that has deteriorated over many years, receiving a diagnosis of a significant health disorder, or strongly worded remarks from others.

When a health seeker experiences a moment of truth, one of two things can happen:

1. He can get *energized* to take action, once and for all.

2. He can *let go* of the goal, and get on with his life.

I'm of the opinion—though I recognize that many health authorities would have my head for saying this—that either of these two possibilities is absolutely positive and should be celebrated. Whether health seekers move this way or that way is immaterial—what matters is that they *move*.

Not too long ago I was coaching a forty-seven-year-old software engineer, Eric, who worked for a company that had hired me for its corporate wellness program. A limitation of the program was that each participant received only six coaching sessions. Despite this, Eric and I quickly established a safe, trusting coaching relationship.

Eric had tried to lose weight on many occasions over the previous ten years. Once, about five years before I met him, he had participated in a weight-loss program called Slim Trimmers and had lost forty-three pounds, but eventually he stopped going, ultimately regaining the weight and then some. On more than one occasion, I suggested to Eric that he return to Slim Trimmers, since he had obtained such good results there the first time and he had a high opinion of them.

At the same time, Eric and I worked on many of the usual things: weekly eating and exercise goals, anticipating obstacles and creative-problem solving, identifying Eric's strengths and building them into his plan, setting boundaries where needed, boosting health confidence—all that good stuff. And yet, each session, I found that Eric did not follow up on his eating and exercise goals, and he did not return to Slim Trimmers. He expressed enthusiasm during our sessions, but afterward he just wouldn't execute.

As I tried to understand, and to help Eric understand, what was going on, he would assume a somewhat self-reproaching tone, saying, "I know, I know. I just need to do it. It's just up to me, and how much I really want it."

Eric was expressing his faith in willpower. We know this to be ill advised, but he could not shake this way of thinking.

In our final session, I asked Eric, "When's the next Slim Trimmers meeting?"

"Tuesday at six o'clock," he replied.

"Go to it," I advised.

"Okay," Eric said.

I'm no psychologist, but sometimes I suspected that Eric used verbal compliance as a means of avoidance.

I asked: "On a scale of one to ten, Eric, how confident are you that you will attend that meeting, where one is not at all confident and ten is absolutely sure?"

"I'd say six," he said. "No, eight. No, seven. I'm a seven. Seven-point-five."

Okay. Here it comes. Recognize that I had discerned in Eric an uncommon readiness for this strong coaching tactic I was about to take.

"Well, here's the thing, Eric," I said. "You've been trying to lose weight for ten years. I hear that it's important to you. You've taken this big step of working with me, a health coach. But beyond that, you take no real action. It seems that every day, you have the intention to get started, yet you don't. Now Slim Trimmers is a great program, and you've gotten results from them in the past. The structure and the social support they offer, based on our conversations, is exactly what you need. The next meeting is Tuesday night. Are you available?"

"Yes."

"Then go. It's time to fish or cut bait. Let this be the litmus test of whether weight loss is really something you're ready to take on right now. So if you don't go, as your coach I'm advising you to let go of your weight-loss goal. Get on with your life. Find another goal that excites you enough and brings you enough joy that you can pursue it with passion. Don't spend the rest of your life planning on losing weight each day. It brings you nothing but grief."

"That's true."

"It doesn't have to be this way, Eric. Understand, I'm not telling you to give up on weight loss. I'm saying either do it, or don't do it. Either way, you'll be better off than living stuck in between."

"Just do it?" he said.

"Just do it, Eric. Or, just don't do it," I told him. "But don't just plan to do it and then not do it. Let Tuesday be your independence day. If you make the commitment and go to Slim Trimmers, then you'll be out of this weight-loss purgatory. If you don't go, take that as a commitment, too, a commitment not to lose weight—at least, not now. And that will free you, as well."

At this point, things clicked for Eric, as he started to get excited about *not* planning to lose weight. And I really could sense a weight being reduced—the weight of the world on Eric's shoulders.

"You know," he said, with more life in his voice than I'd heard since our coaching sessions began, "I've even heard that some people only lose weight when they stop trying."

"Well, I've certainly known that to be the case, Eric," I acknowledged. But I had to be honest with him: "However, there's a trap there. If you stop trying to lose weight with the idea that you will lose weight because you've stopped trying, then you haven't really stopped trying, and the whole thing falls apart."

"I think I understood that," he kidded.

"What I *have* seen happen, though, is that when people stop running in circles with weight-loss planning—or any health change—they can put that energy into something that brings them more joy. Once they have that joy in their lives, they may already have achieved what they were hoping to achieve through weight loss, or the joy may be just the prerequisite they need to launch a successful weight-loss effort, once and for all."

"I get it. Thank you, Bob."

Admittedly, if Eric had been advised by a physician to lose weight, or if he had high blood pressure or diabetes or was extremely obese, I may not have been able to take this strong approach. But that was not the case. Still, you may ask, "Isn't being overweight a health risk in and of itself? So isn't it irresponsible to ignore it?"

Yes, being overweight is a health risk. It can lead to heart disease and diabetes. Overweight people are discriminated against and may lack self-esteem. If you are overweight and you can reduce your weight, then do it. But the fact is, not every person can do it at any given time.

Moments of truth are not moments of resignation. Recall that in our conversations, Eric sounded resigned *before* his moment of truth, whereas he became quite animated afterward. Confronting the truth about a long-standing, unrealized goal is not quitting; on the contrary, it's a giant leap forward.

What's more, the point of a moment of truth is not necessarily to let go of a goal, but to let go of your attachment to an *unrealized* goal. After a moment of truth, many health seekers dig in and make the change. Others dig out and redirect their energy elsewhere.

And Eric? He sent me a holiday card last year. He wrote that he had been participating in Slim Trimmers for the past six months, had already lost twenty-six pounds, and felt better than ever.

MIND YOUR CHANGE

Moments of truth are opportunities for growth, but they can be quite difficult. Sometimes they are internally generated when health seekers encounter a truth they may not care to confront, such as an unkind comment they overhear, a photo of themselves from long ago, getting out of breath while climbing a flight of stairs, or finding that they don't have the upper body strength to lift their child or grandchild.

Think back over the past month. Have you experienced any of these moments but been so engrossed in the anguish that you failed to notice the possibility?

Be vigilant for moments of truth. You see now that they represent not only wonderful flashes of insight, but powerful opportunities to transform negative experiences into positive, life-affirming milestones.

LIFE BALANCE REVISITED

Eᴠᴇʀ since Dr. Halbert Dunn proposed in the 1950s that "high-level wellness" encompasses the physical, emotional, psychological, and spiritual realms of our lives—and not just the absence of disease—wellness know-it-alls have spurred health seekers to establish balance among these various realms. Sometimes they divide them differently to include your work, finances, environment, relationships, and so forth.

Nowhere has the cry for balance been louder than in coaching circles. We coaches have taken the position, perhaps paradoxically, that in order to excel in one area of wellness you first must establish balance in all realms, without getting hung up in any particular one. This point of view represents a challenge for health coaches when we encounter the client who, say, loves physical activity and hikes for three hours a day. Should we advise such a client to exercise less so he can devote more time to his job or to spirituality? Let's come back to this question in a moment.

In the early days of my own business Web site, I wrote, "It's all about balance." But I've changed that. It may very well be all about balance, but not necessarily as balance has been understood in the conventional wellness sense—that is, giving equal attention and energy to each aspect of wellness.

If a balanced life appeals to you, recognize that balance can take many forms and that it fits different people in different ways. Here are five insights on balance that will help you find the best fit for you:

- *Great people throughout world history did not have balance, in the conventional sense, in their lives.* Van Gogh, Einstein, and Martin Luther King Jr. led lives with a singular focus. Civilization has always depended upon people without conventional balance to spark the most revolutionary improvements in our society. In a way, they balance out the rest of us, on the grandest of scales.

- *Striving to afford equal attention to each of the realms of wellness is often a recipe for mediocrity.* This is acceptable to some people, but not to others.

- *The universe maintains a natural balance.* You are part of it, no matter what your date book looks like.

- *Balance exists in your life in the present moment.* If you seek balance, take a few deep breaths and clear your mind of thoughts, memories, plans, and overpowering emotions. After you let go of these, you'll find it: Balance!

- *Realize the distinctions: balance, passion, and chaos.* You may feel that chaos in your life is driving you bonkers and yearn for balance. On the other hand, you may have conventional balance in your life and yearn for passion.

Another important distinction involves compulsiveness. Consider the client mentioned earlier who hikes three hours a day. Is he compulsive, or just passionate? We don't have enough information to formulate an opinion. I want to know if he likes what he's doing. Are there signs that other activities or people in his life are suffering as a result of his commitment? Is he injuring himself? And is he "at-choice" in the matter?

Compulsive or passionate? It's a question that comes up frequently with health seekers who exercise several hours a day, or with others whose dietary regimen may at first seem extreme. But we can't be too quick to draw conclusions. A lot of these folks are just exceptionally passionate...and incredibly fit. If the behavior *is* compulsive, then the assistance of a mental health professional probably is in order.

This topic of balance is one of those rare instances when I don't have any sage counsel for you. You must find your own way here. But I hope I have given you, if not a roadmap, at least some attractive choices for a destination.

M IND Y OUR C HANGE

Use a paper plate and a pencil to make a pie chart. Draw straight lines from the center to the edge so you're creating several "slices," with each slice representing one of the realms of wellness: physical, mental, spiritual, environment, or whatever you think belongs. Make each slice proportionate to the amount of time and energy you devote to each realm. Now find the exact center of the paper plate, spin the plate on your fingertip and stand on your head—okay, not really. It's just an analogy to make a point: Your life can be balanced even when the activities in it are not.

DOES YOUR JOB MAKE YOU SICK?

SEVERAL years back I was working as a consultant for a national insurance company that wanted to institute a worksite health-promotion program for its employees. We were in the development stages of the program, and many of the employees at the headquarters office had gotten to know me via meetings and informational sessions. One morning, as I was walking down a long aisle between rows of stark beige cubicles, a middle-aged female employee rolled her chair back to block my path and asked, "Can I talk to you for a minute?"

"Sure," I said. There wasn't really space for another body in her cube, but I took a step toward its entryway to give her my full attention.

She introduced herself to me as Betty Rose. "I just think it's ironic," she said, casting furtive glances left and right to see if she was being overheard, "that the company is going to all this effort to help us lead healthier lives, when in fact the main thing that stands in the way of my wellness is this job."

It was a compelling point, and one that I've heard repeatedly from employees who work for companies where wellness programs are being developed. Many employees perceive that the stress of their jobs renders it virtually impossible to lead a healthy lifestyle. A recent run on books with such titles as *Toxic Co-Workers, Working Wounded,* and *Work Abuse* confirms this image of the workplace as a debilitating wasteland.

As I chatted with Betty Rose, who worked in the company's call center handling customer inquiries and complaints, she really opened up about her job and its impact on her health. "This call center used to have fifty people in it. Now, due to downsizing, it has eighteen. But has the volume of calls gone down? No. It's gone up by 20 percent. Customers have to wait on hold longer and longer. By the time they actually get to speak with me, they're already fuming. I'm supposed to take a higher volume of calls, yet give full attention to each caller. That's contradictory—flat-out impossible!" Betty Rose was getting riled now, venting steam that clearly had been pent up for a long time.

"They've put in this new computer system, and it's a total dog," she continued. "Now I have to go to four screens to deal with an inquiry, compared to the old system where I only needed one screen. I've complained to my boss about this, but he just gives me some song and dance about all the great data reports the new system generates. The company has been cutting back on the claims it will cover, so there's not much I can do to appease most of these customers who are complaining. My job is strictly to recite policy. And when some of the customers complain that an exception should be made for them because their situation doesn't really fit what the policy was made for, they're usually right. But I'm not allowed to make that exception. And I know that in some of these cases the exception would actually save the company money, but I'm still not allowed to make the exception. More and more of the other staff are calling in sick, and now I'm getting called in to work on weekends or evenings. My family is starting to forget what I look like. And what do I get for all this? Probably laid off in the next round of downsizing. I am so burnt out and fed up, that to hear the company invite me to a workshop on Balancing Work and Family, or encourage me to start a fitness program when I have no time, is absolutely ridiculous."

Thanks to Betty Rose and a few others who shared their feelings, we were able to collaborate with Human Resources to promote several changes in the way things were run. But I must admit it was an uphill battle, mostly because the lion's share of the company's executive team was too preoccupied with the bravado of "belt-tightening" to look at the big picture—or at themselves and their own styles of leadership. The wellness program turned out to be little more than a bone thrown the employees' way, and it saddens me to acknowledge that it did little to evoke real change among the staff of this troubled organization, which eventually tightened its belt right out of existence.

The primary reason that worksite wellness programs in the United States have failed to live up to their original promise—building a healthier, more productive workforce and containing health-care costs—is that these programs have focused on individual health behaviors with total disregard for the maladies and health risks that are intrinsic to the organization itself. CEOs can be sold on the idea that their employees' behaviors must change, but they refuse to assess their *own* leadership behaviors and the manner in which they treat those employees.

Over the past thirty years, a strong body of scientific evidence has emerged supporting the theory that employee health is driven primarily by organizational dynamics, and not simply by individual behaviors.

Stress, which has been linked to the full gamut of physical ailments—from back pain to heart disease and even gastrointestinal disorders—is one of the greatest occupational health hazards. But there's more to stress than meets the eye. Fast-paced, challenging, intense jobs, for example, do not necessarily lead to harmful stress.

In the workplace, harmful stress is a product of having a lot expected of you and having little control over it. This has become known as the demand-control model of workplace health. Betty Rose is a perfect example of an employee with high demand and low control. The company demanded that she increase her productivity despite diminishing resources, yet she wasn't granted the control to make exceptions or to have input into the computer system. This type of control is also known as "decisional latitude"—the capacity to make decisions affecting a wide breadth of an employee's work.

The effects of high demands and low control are further confounded by "psychosocial" shortcomings in the workplace—including a lack of both emotional and technical support from coworkers, as well as supervisors.

A different but equally important view of stress in the workplace points to the relationship between employees' efforts and their potential rewards. Intensely demanding work along with, for example, minimal job security and few career-advancement opportunities, leads to harmful job stress. One can't help but speculate on what the implications of the effort-reward model are for Americans, such as Betty Rose, who are working harder than ever for rewards that pale compared to other wealthy, industrialized societies.

A recent report by the Economic Policy Institute revealed that today the average middle-income, two-parent family is working 660 more hours per year—the equivalent of sixteen more weeks—than they did twenty years ago. "America remains the reigning workaholic nation," the report noted. "The average worker worked 1,877 hours in 2000—more than in any other rich, industrialized country. At the same time, Americans reap fewer benefits for these extra hours, whether in the form of more vacation or holiday time or paid leave time of the sort provided by almost every other advanced economy."

A Finnish study recently investigated stress due to *high-demand and low-control* jobs and to *high-effort and low-reward* jobs. The research showed that both kinds of stress *doubled* employee risk of cardiovascular death. They also were linked to such health risks as elevated cholesterol levels and excessive weight gain.

If dysfunctional organizations lead to stress and stress leads to illness, then is your job making you sick? You bet it is. And an employee brown-bag workshop on Balancing Work and Family is not going to make you better.

The demand-control model and the lesser-known effort-reward model reflect the view that work stress and health outcomes are not simply a result of personal behaviors. Even the United States Government has come to support this premise and has begun to promote it to Wall Street and Main Street, where it has yet to take hold. While acknowledging that stress-management programs targeting employee behaviors play an important supporting role, the U.S. National Institute for Occupational Safety and Health (NIOSH) takes the following stand: "As a general rule, actions to reduce job stress should give top priority to organizational change to improve working conditions."

What type of organizational change? NIOSH recommends that employers:

- Ensure that the workload is in line with workers' capabilities and resources.

- Design jobs to provide meaning, stimulation, and opportunities for workers to use their skills.

- Clearly define workers' roles and responsibilities.

- Give workers opportunities to participate in decisions and actions affecting their jobs.

- Provide opportunities for social interaction among workers.

- Establish work schedules that are compatible with demands and responsibilities outside the job.

NIOSH takes to task companies that insist that stress is a necessary evil if they wish to remain profitable. The agency points out that stressful working conditions are actually associated with increased absenteeism, tardiness, and employee turnover—all of which adversely affect a company's bottom line.

Robert Karasek, an expert in industrial systems and psychology, developed and popularized the demand-control model throughout the 1970s and 1980s. His theories were not a mere exercise in academics, but were applied in many industrial settings. Ultimately, they redefined organizational theory and occupational health in Scandinavian countries with dramatic, well-documented results.

Karasek argues that even typical smoking-cessation programs, which target individual smokers, underestimate the role of stress related to poor job design. Such stress, he notes, may well be at the root of employee smoking.

But can jobs and corporations really be restructured to create a healthier environment for employees? And even if such changes do improve health, would it be at the expense of productivity?

Karasek has documented many examples—in a variety of business sectors—of employers who restructured work and, as a result, improved employee health and *increased* productivity. One such example is Volvo, the Swedish car manufacturer, which instituted a work redesign program companywide, from assembly-line workers to executives.

One Volvo work group was studied intensively. The group implemented far-reaching changes that included a more facilitative management style, job redesign, a less confrontational role for union leadership, and a smoking-cessation program.

Two years later, studies showed a decrease in the incidence of employee depression and fatigue, stress, and gastrointestinal symptoms. Smoking rates plummeted. At the same time, productivity improved measurably: Customer demands were handled more effectively, employee motivation improved, profits linked to the group increased, and the employees' workload increased moderately, despite the reports of decreased stress.

I have found, in my own experience, that American companies' failings in this type of effort reflect our skewed vision of how a team is supposed to function.

In the 1980s and 1990s, team-building became another buzzword in corporate America, and suddenly we all were showing up at the water cooler with coffee mugs—graciously distributed to us by our buddies in Human Resources—sporting the slogan "There Is No 'I' In Team." Well, that about says it, doesn't it?

I've never visited a Scandinavian country, but I've been told that most Americans would be shocked to witness how much latitude individual employees there—at all levels—have in making major decisions.

But in the U.S., teamwork had the opposite effect. After all, "There is no 'I' in team." As a result of this misguided notion of teamwork, many American employees became disempowered. Instead of encouraging individual decision making, the message was: Don't make a move without consulting everyone else.

Thinking about switching the toilet paper in the staff bathrooms to a softer brand? Call a team meeting. The team can then assign who will do the price comparison, who will research ply, who will set up a system for measuring individual sheet size and sheets-per-roll, who will contact any other teams that may require "buy-in," and who will launch the "roll-out." If there ever is one, that is.

There may be no "I" in team, but corporate execs would be well served to remember that there *is* an "I" in decision—more than one, in fact. Decisional latitude and fully functional teams can co-exist.

If you are in a position of clout, I urge you to further investigate the demand-control model and steer your organization toward promoting decisional latitude at every level. If you believe you are not in a position of clout . . . well, that's the problem right there.

Be aware that decisional latitude applies to *all* employees, including line workers and manual laborers. Work with your union or coworkers to campaign for increased decisional latitude. Scandinavia had its Industrial Democratization Movement; perhaps it's time for an Industrial Democratization Revolution in the U.S.

Each employee brings great potential and gifts to the workplace. It's in the best interest of not only employee health but also organizational health to put those gifts to work.

MIND YOUR CHANGE

Research has shown that if you believe your job undermines your health, chances are good that it will. According to studies, you are likely to perceive your job as deleterious to your health if you:

- Have limited control in your work life.

- Work at least one night, or more than forty-five hours, per week.

- Earn more—that's right, *more*—than ten dollars per hour.

- Tend not to be outgoing.

On the other hand, you are more likely to perceive your job as having a *positive* influence on your health if you:

- Are older.

- Are a member of a minority group.

- Have less education.

- Have more control.

- Are self-employed.

- Hold a job that has greater physical demands, entails less repetitive work, and requires greater intelligence.

Take a look at this list of job qualities. Obviously, there are many that you can't do anything about. But some you can. Determine what actions you can take to help you shift your own perception of how your work affects your health. If it appears that you don't have any choice over any of these aspects of your work life, revisit the "Choose Well" chapter in this handbook.

THE LIFE CYCLE OF CHANGE: HOW LONG DOES IT TAKE?

WHEN you make a health change, such as eating better, exercising more, reducing stress, or even something as seemingly minor as switching from whole milk to nonfat, you tend to think of that change as taking place at a particular time—tomorrow, New Year's Day, next month...whenever you promise yourself you're going to take action. In fact, your changes usually are more of an evolution rather than a revolution; that is, you go through a process, a series of distinct stages.

Behavioral researchers led by James Prochaska have defined six specific stages of change and have shown that health seekers are much more likely to be successful if they pass through each stage, rather than skipping one or more. For most changes you've already made, you almost certainly passed through these stages, even if it seemed as if you changed all at once.

The specific stages of change are:

1. *Precontemplation.* This is the stage in which you are not even thinking about changing.

2. *Contemplation.* You're considering changing a health habit (starting a good one or stopping a bad one) within the next six months.

3. *Preparation.* You're committed to initiating a change within the next thirty days.

4. *Action.* You are actively changing your behavior.

5. *Maintenance.* You have made the change; now you strive to prevent relapse.

6. *Termination.* You are no longer even tempted by your former health behavior.

I call this process the Life Cycle of Change because the model is circular, not linear. While most health seekers start as precontemplators, once you have entered the process you can exit and then re-enter at any stage you've already completed.

Stages-of-change theory owes much to the other change theories that it integrates and builds upon. For example, many of the beliefs that bog down precontemplators are comparable to those that limit health-program participation in Hochbaum's Health Belief Model, which was cited in the "Believe This" chapter of this book. What's more, for each stage of change there's a correlating level of health confidence, which is based on Banduras's self-efficacy theory. And finally, progress through the early stages of change is largely mediated by the health seeker's assessment of the pros and cons of changing, a model for decision making that was brought to notoriety in the mid-1970s by psychologists Irving Janis and Leon Mann. But no one theory has painted a picture of the health change process as vividly and precisely as Stages of Change.

Many health seekers have heard that it takes a certain time period—generally defined as six weeks, eight weeks, or twelve weeks—for a new behavior to become a habit (in this context, "habit" means that the behavior has become effortless). Studies of the Maintenance stage and the Termination stage—the last two components in the Stages of Change model—answer the question "How long does it take for a new behavior to become a habit?" You might not like the answer, but your chances of success are greater if you at least know what the answer is.

First, let's get clear about what each of these two stages represents:

- In the Maintenance stage, you actively work to avoid relapsing back to your old behavior, but you don't work as hard as you did when you were first making your change. Health confidence is on the rise.

- In the Termination stage, there is zero temptation and 100 percent health confidence. The Termination stage is what most people are talking about when they refer to a new behavior becoming a habit or second nature.

In effect, the question "How long does it take for a new behavior to become a habit?" is really asking "How long does it take to go from the Maintenance stage to the Termination stage?" Leading behaviorists have disavowed the Termination stage, claiming that no one ever reaches it. Of course that's not true. Most health seekers have reached termination for at least one behavior. But ironically, the new behavior has come to feel so natural to you that you forget to give yourself credit for it. If you've worn eyeglasses all your life, you can have them on all day without even momentarily being aware of them. The same is true for health habits: You have worn certain behaviors for so long, you no longer are conscious of them. That is true Termination.

For example, many health seekers have chosen to stop eating red meat and are not the least bit tempted to go back to it. Others have switched from whole milk to reduced-fat milk, and now find whole milk revolting. I even know health seekers who, in midlife, started flossing their teeth daily and certainly were in no danger of discontinuing this often overlooked yet vital health practice. These health seekers reached Termination.

These same health seekers, however, also made health changes for which they did *not* reach Termination, but instead remained in the Maintenance stage. For instance, most health seekers who switched from whole milk to low-fat milk ultimately sought to reduce fat throughout their diets, yet are constantly tempted by ice cream sundaes, juicy steaks, or french fries. Because they actively work to resist temptation, they are considered to be in Maintenance and may never reach Termination.

Perhaps now you have figured out how long the Maintenance stage lasts—that is, how long it takes for a new behavior to become a habit, with no special effort required. Prochaska estimated that for many health behaviors, Maintenance lasts from six months to about five years. But even Prochaska has come to de-emphasize the Termination stage altogether, because for many people dealing with prevalent health behaviors—such as exercise and weight management—he has found that the realistic goal may be a *lifetime* of Maintenance. Ouch.

I'm not quite ready to let go of the Termination stage, however. I find that all health seekers have reached Termination for some change they have made. And those kinds of changes—whether or not they seem like life-changing transformations—serve as a model for what is possible.

It's safe to say, then, that the length of the Maintenance stage ultimately depends on the individual and on the specific change that's being made. While this may not be as comforting as the belief that you're on easy street once you've practiced your new behavior for six, eight, or twelve weeks, it will behoove you in the long run to enter into your change with both eyes wide open. If you naively expect that you will be free and clear, for example, after six weeks, then you may succumb to complacency at that time and prematurely let your guard down. On the other hand, if you initiate change with the understanding that it may require a lifelong effort, you are more likely to enter into it with the greatest possible commitment, and having called to action all available resources.

Research has shown that in the Maintenance stage, relapse is most likely to occur when you are experiencing emotional distress—feeling sad, anxious, lonely, angry, or bored (whereas, in the Termination stage, even these difficult states won't lead to a setback). The bottom line is, when you are in the Maintenance stage, be vigilant for troubling emotions, and be sure to build extra self-care into your life. Avoid volunteering for stressful projects, take vacations, try yoga, get massages, stay clear of your in-laws, listen to calming music, spend time with your pet, take walks in beautiful surroundings.

Prochaska's studies revealed that health seekers almost always have setbacks. But for most behaviors, they rarely relapse all the way back to Precontemplation. Most return to contemplating or preparing for another serious attempt at action.

This is one of the main reasons that awareness of the stages of change is invaluable. Typically, when you relapse you might be inclined to think *"Yikes, now I have to start all over from the beginning."* The prospect could be so daunting that it intimidates you from getting back in the saddle. But now you know that, after relapse, you're not really starting all over again. You are still in the saddle. And all you need to do is gently spur your pony on. No nags, please.

Now, giddy-up.

MIND YOUR CHANGE

If the Maintenance stage can last a lifetime, then you probably are in the Maintenance stage right now for a change you've already made. Identify at least one of these changes. What circumstances are coming up in your life that may cause you emotional distress and potentially lead to relapse? House guests? A project deadline? Upcoming holidays? Take action today to manage these circumstances or your reactions to them. Rearrange plans if you can, make an appointment for a massage, or schedule whatever activity will bring you the most peace. Remember, you hold the reins.

HEALTHMATE COACHING

$\mathbf{W}$ITH today's emphasis on health, you are likely to encounter in your everyday life countless health seekers who are trying to adopt good health practices or dispose of bad ones. Perhaps they wish to improve their eating habits or start an exercise program. Maybe they want to reduce stress or to quit smoking. Do you think you can help them? You bet you can. No matter who you are or what your background is, you can be a "healthmate coach." Your healthmate may be a coworker, a friend, a spouse, or even your long-lost cousin from Buffalo.

Often potential healthmate coaches are reluctant to offer their help, fearful that they'll be perceived as nagging. This concern is well founded. Healthmate coaches whose motives are driven primarily by their own needs or who don't have a handle on coaching skills probably *are* nagging.

So when you first consider coaching a healthmate, start by examining your motives. Are you driven by your own judgment that your healthmate would be better off by changing? Or worse, that *you* would somehow benefit from it? Or is your desire to help based on a sincere wish to give support where it's needed? If your motivation is rooted in the spirit of giving, you needn't worry about nagging.

Once your motives are clear, get started. Here are twelve key strategies for a healthmate coach:

1. "Enroll" your healthmates in coaching. Get their permission and "buy in."

2. Understand what stage of change your healthmates are in and support them accordingly.

3. Help your healthmates discover their possibility.

4. Help your healthmates develop an action plan with both short- and long-term goals.

5. Celebrate your healthmates' actions.

6. Be assertive, as appropriate. Hold your healthmates accountable to sticking with the plan.

7. Listen to your healthmates' concerns about their action plans. Endorse them for good insights and strong efforts. But also point out when excuses are just that: excuses.

8. Acknowledge your healthmates' strengths, such as perseverance, planning, or enthusiasm.

9. Boost your healthmates' health confidence by exploring past self-improvements, by modeling good health habits, and by providing unconditional support and encouragement.

10. Accept that you are not responsible for your healthmates' success or failure. Your healthmates do the work—and live with the consequences, good or bad.

11. Recognize that many health practices, such as substance abuse, require professional care, not healthmate coaching.

12. Direct your healthmates to useful resources, such as books, Web sites, and organizations.

Rest assured that you do not have to be an expert or have specific experience with a health practice in order to coach a healthmate. After all, your job is not to diagnose or to treat, but to be a partner in change. And if you reflect upon your life, on successful shifts you have made, you will find that you have learned a great deal about personal change, and that your experience in this arena is unlimited.

MIND YOUR CHANGE
In several previous "Mind Your Change" activities, you were asked to reflect on changes you have already made. Now, think of one person in your life who is trying to make one of these same changes. Flip back through this book and choose five strategies you can share with this prospective healthmate. Strategize how you might "enroll" your healthmate in the coaching process without being a nag. Whose agenda will be served by entry into a healthmate coaching relationship—your healthmate's, or yours?

Afterword

In *The Health Seeker's Handbook,* you have read a lot about how beliefs can shape the actions you choose to take. I'd like to leave you with a word about my own beliefs, which have seen me through many personal health changes and have influenced the manner in which I've coached countless health seekers to make positive changes beyond what they had ever imagined possible.

I believe that each of us is endowed with a spark of universal power. And if you take care of that spark, it will become a flame.

I believe that you are *not:*

- Your weight.

- Your fitness level.

- Your stress.

- Your behaviors.

These are a *part* of your experience, but they are not who you are. When you are mindful of these aspects of your life, you will be able to modify them—if you choose—naturally and without resistance.

My closing wish for you is to get better acquainted with the spark inside of you, to let it grow into a flame, to reveal that flame to others, and to bask in its warmth and light.

SELECTED BIBLIOGRAPHY

American College of Sports Medicine. *ACSM's Guidelines for Exercise Testing and Prescription.* 6th ed. Baltimore: Lippincott, Williams, and Wilkins, 2000.

Brown, K.W. and Ryan, R.M. "The Benefits of Being Present: Mindfulness and Its Role in Psychological Well-Being." *Journal of Personality and Social Psychology* 84 (2003): 822-48.

Dunn, H. *High Level Wellness.* Arlington, VA: R.W. Beatty, 1961.

Economic Policy Institute. *The State of Working America, 2002-03.* Ithaca, NY: Cornell University Press, 2003.

Elder, J.P., Ayala, M.A., and Harris, S. "Theories and Intervention Approaches to Health-Behavior Change in Primary Care." *American Journal of Preventive Medicine* 17 (1999): 275-84.

Ettner, S.L. and Grzywacz, J.G. "Workers' Perceptions of How Jobs Affect Health: A Social Ecological Perspective." *Journal of Occupational Health Psychology* 6 (2001): 101-13.

Glanz, K., Lewis, M.F., and Rimer, B.K., eds. *Health Behavior and Health Education: Theory, Research, and Practice.* 3rd ed. San Francisco: Jossey-Bass, 2002.

Grodstein, F., et al. "Three-Year Follow-up of Participants in a Commercial Weight Loss Program. Can you keep it off?" *Archives of Internal Medicine* 156 (1996):1302-1306.

Hu, F.B., et al. "Television Watching and Other Sedentary Behaviors in Relation to Risk of Obesity and Type 2 Diabetes Mellitus in Women." *JAMA* 14 (2003):1785-1791.

Institute of Medicine. *Dietary Reference Intakes for Energy, Carbohydrate, Fiber, Fat, Fatty Acids, Cholesterol, Protein, and Amino Acids (Macronutrients).* Washington, DC: National Academies Press, 2002.

Karasek, R. and Therell, T. *Healthy Work: Stress, Productivity, and the Reconstruction of Working Life.* New York: Basic Books, 1990.

Kivimki, M., et al. "Work Stress and Risk of Cardiovascular Mortality: Prospective Cohort Study of Industrial Employees." *British Medical Journal* 325 (2002): 857.

Nigg, C.R., Allegrante, J.P., and Ory, M. "Theory-Comparison and Multiple-Behavior Research: Common Themes Advancing Health Behavior Research." *Health Education Research* 17 (2002): 670-679.

Patton, R.W., et al. *Implementing Health Fitness Programs.* Champaign, IL: Human Kinetics, 1986.

Prochaska, J.O. and Velicer, W.F. "The Transtheoretical Model of Health Behavior Change." *American Journal of Health Promotion* 12 (1997): 38-48.

Sidney, S., et al. "Television Viewing and Cardiovascular Risk Factors in Young Adults: The CARDIA Study." *Annals of Epidemiology* 6 (1996):154-159.

Sauter, S. *Stress...At Work.* National Institute for Occupational Safety and Health. Department of Health and Human Services (NIOSH) Publication No. 99-101. 1999.

Wing, R.R. and Hill, J.O. "Successful Weight Loss Maintenance." *Annual Review of Nutrition* 21 (2001): 323-41.

Wing, R.R., et al. "Behavioral Research in Diabetes: Lifestyle Changes Related to Obesity, Eating Behavior, and Physical Activity." *Diabetes Care* 24 (2001): 117-123.

World Health Organization Regional Office for Europe. *Ottawa Charter for Health Promotion, 1986.* WHO Web site.

Recommended Reading

You can purchase these books at discount prices via the Web site of The Center for Personal Health Coaching at www.healthcoach4u.com (this address is subject to change):

The Art of Getting Well by David Spero (Alameda, Calif.: Hunter House Publishers, 2002). Spero, a registered nurse who was diagnosed with multiple sclerosis more than twelve years ago, advocates many of the same methods that are promoted here in *The Health Seeker's Handbook.* But as a clinician and a leading health coach, he distinctly tailors his insightful and practical book to readers living with chronic disease.

The Art of Possibility by Rosamund Stone Zander and Benjamin Zander (Boston: Harvard Business School Press, 2000). The authors don't just describe, but demonstrate, how our lives can be transformed by removing our filters and seeing the previously unimaginable universe of possibilities that lies before us.

Changing for Good by James Prochaska, John Norcross, and Carlo DiClemente (New York: Avon Books, 1994). Prochaska has published volumes of scientific literature. In this book, he translates his findings and theories on Stages of Change into a system that any health seeker can use.

Coaching by John Flaherty (Boston: Butterworth-Heinemann, 1999). An excellent primer on coaching techniques that integrates a scholarly approach with hands-on practicality. Includes a brief but stinging refutation of the use of behaviorism in coaching. An important text for coaches or anyone thinking of becoming a coach.

Eat, Drink, and Be Healthy by Walter Willett (New York: Simon and Schuster, 2001). The best book on healthy eating. Willett sorts out, without any agenda other than sharing the truth, fact from fiction regarding fats, carbohydrates, and protein, as well as supplements, fluid intake, and weight maintenance.

Full Catastrophe Living by Jon Kabat-Zinn (New York: Dell Publishing, 1990). The ultimate, scientifically based resource on how to evoke stress reduction and healing through the practice of mindfulness.

Guide to Stress Reduction, revised edition, by L. John Mason (Berkeley, CA: Celestial Arts, 2001). Offers such a broad array of techniques that you are sure to find several that suit you regardless of your particular circumstances. It runs the gamut, including deep breathing, autogenics, progressive relaxation, exercise, biofeedback, desensitization, and nutrition. Valuable new sections include explorations of "specific ailments and stress reduction" and "stress reduction in business."

Making Peace with Food by Susan Kano (New York: Harper and Row, 1989). An excellent instruction manual for freeing yourself from the diet and weight obsession. Kano sorts through the stigmas and frustration associated with overweight without invalidating readers' intentions to lose weight. She offers a ton of practical advice and techniques on how to achieve weight goals while maintaining a positive self-image.

The Miracle of Mindfulness by Thich Nhat Hanh (Boston: Beacon Press, 1999). Zen Master Thich Nhat Hanh, who was nominated for a Nobel Peace Prize by Martin Luther King Jr., offers simple instructions for mindfulness and meditation.

Peace Is Every Step by Thich Nhat Hanh (New York: Bantam, 1992). This beautiful book about mindfulness has changed the lives of thousands, perhaps millions, of people. It may change yours.

Take Time for Your Life by Cheryl Richardson (New York: Broadway Books, 1999). This is the book that put coaching on the map. Richardson distills classic coaching techniques into a format you can use for your own self-development. Especially useful for those who respond to high-energy, unrelenting positivism.

Taming Your Gremlin by Richard Carson (New York: HarperCollins, 2003). An entertaining and wildly insightful book about the internal voices that hold us back in life, and how to quiet them.

Wherever You Go, There You Are by Jon Kabat-Zinn (New York: Hyperion, 1994). A best-selling primer on mindfulness, especially appealing to those who prefer a secular approach.

Zen Mind, Beginner's Mind by Shunryu Suzuki (New York: Weatherhill, 1980). The seminal treatise on Beginner's Mind. You will need to be a bit of a zen fan to appreciate this book fully.

Printed in the United States
29684LVS00001B/413